Dr. med. Sophia K. Johnson, MD
Dipl.-Biol. Jana Pastuschek, M. sc.

PLACENTA POWER

Stadelmann

Dr. med. Sophia K. Johnson, MD
Dipl.-Biol. Jana Pastuschek, M. sc.

PLACENTA POWER

Stadelmann

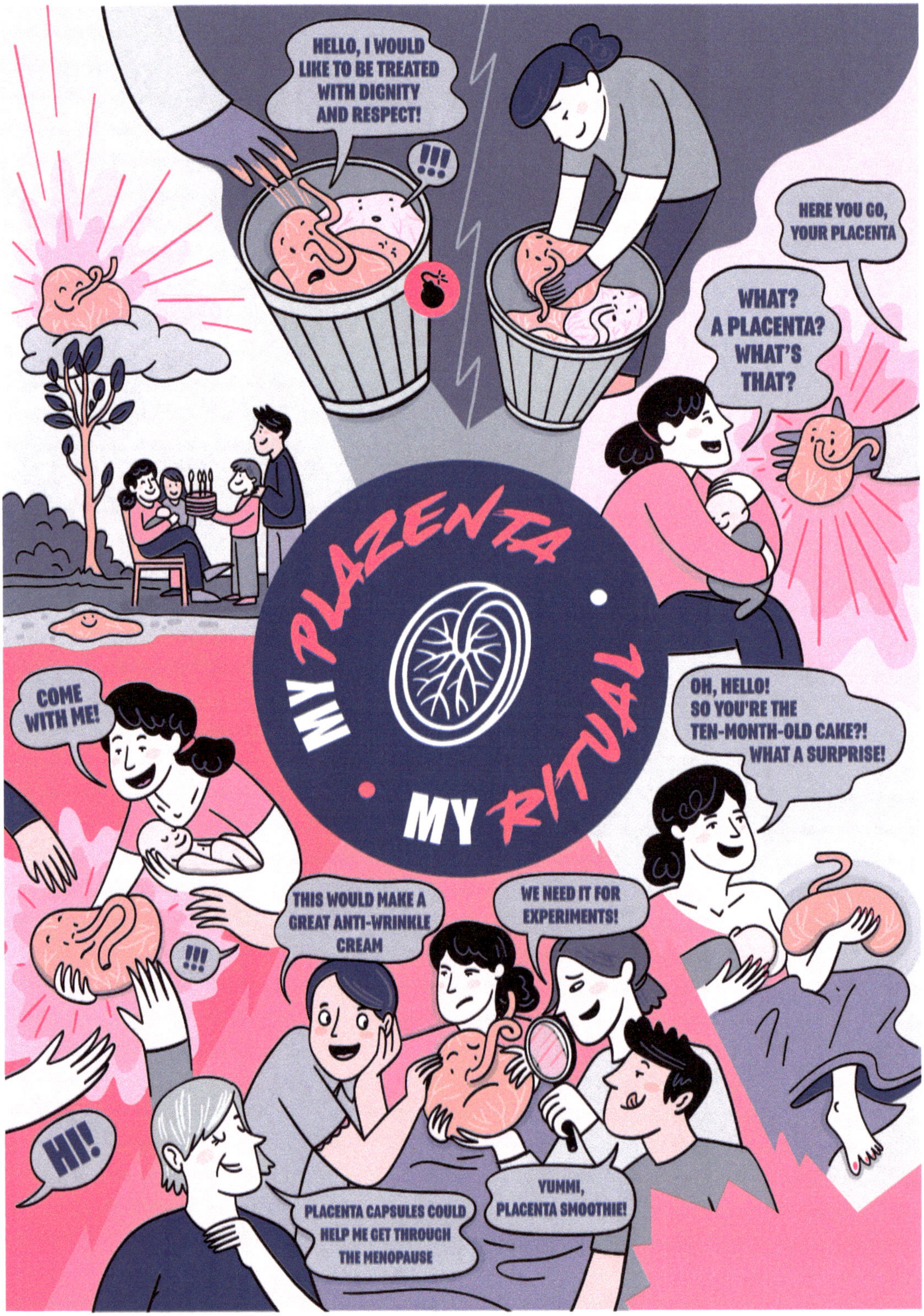
HELLO, I WOULD LIKE TO BE TREATED WITH DIGNITY AND RESPECT!
!!!
HERE YOU GO, YOUR PLACENTA
WHAT? A PLACENTA? WHAT'S THAT?
MY PLAZENTA
MY RITUAL
OH, HELLO! SO YOU'RE THE TEN-MONTH-OLD CAKE?! WHAT A SURPRISE!
COME WITH ME!
!!!
THIS WOULD MAKE A GREAT ANTI-WRINKLE CREAM
WE NEED IT FOR EXPERIMENTS!
HI!
YUMMI, PLACENTA SMOOTHIE!
PLACENTA CAPSULES COULD HELP ME GET THROUGH THE MENOPAUSE

1st edition 2023
978-3-96914-037-6

Nesso 8, 87487 Wiggensbach
www.stadelmann-verlag.de
bestellung@stadelmann-verlag.de

German Proofreading: Mariette Franz (www.mariette-franz.de)
Production: Eberl & Koesel Studio, Kempten
English translation: Dr. med. Sophia Johnson
Proofreading of the English translation: Professor Sheila Dickson,
University of Glasgow
Lecturing: Professor Sheila Dickson, University of Glasgow

IMPORTANT NOTE

The ideas, methods and suggestions in this book represent the opinions and experiences of the authors. They have been compiled by the authors to the best of their knowledge and checked with the greatest possible care. However, they are no substitute for personal and medical advice. Each reader remains responsible for his or her own actions. The information provided here should never be used as the sole source for health-related decisions. It should not be used as a basis for independent diagnoses or for starting, changing or stopping treatment of illnesses. Readers are urged to contact appropriate medical professionals when making such medical decisions. Accordingly, the authors are not responsible for any injuries or adverse consequences arising from any suggestions or advice given in this book.

Additionally, this book contains references to websites and books over whose content the authors had no role in either producing or influencing. Therefore, the authors are not responsible for any injuries or other adverse consequences arising from reliance by readers upon any such websites or books.

The manuscript of this book was written by Sophia Johnson. Jana Pastuschek was involved in the lecturing- and review process and contributed following sub-chapters: The toxic Placenta, The phylogenetic origin of the placenta and parts of The placenta as a research object, Hotly debated: Placenta and microbiome and Introduction to our placenta universe.

TABLE OF CONTENTS

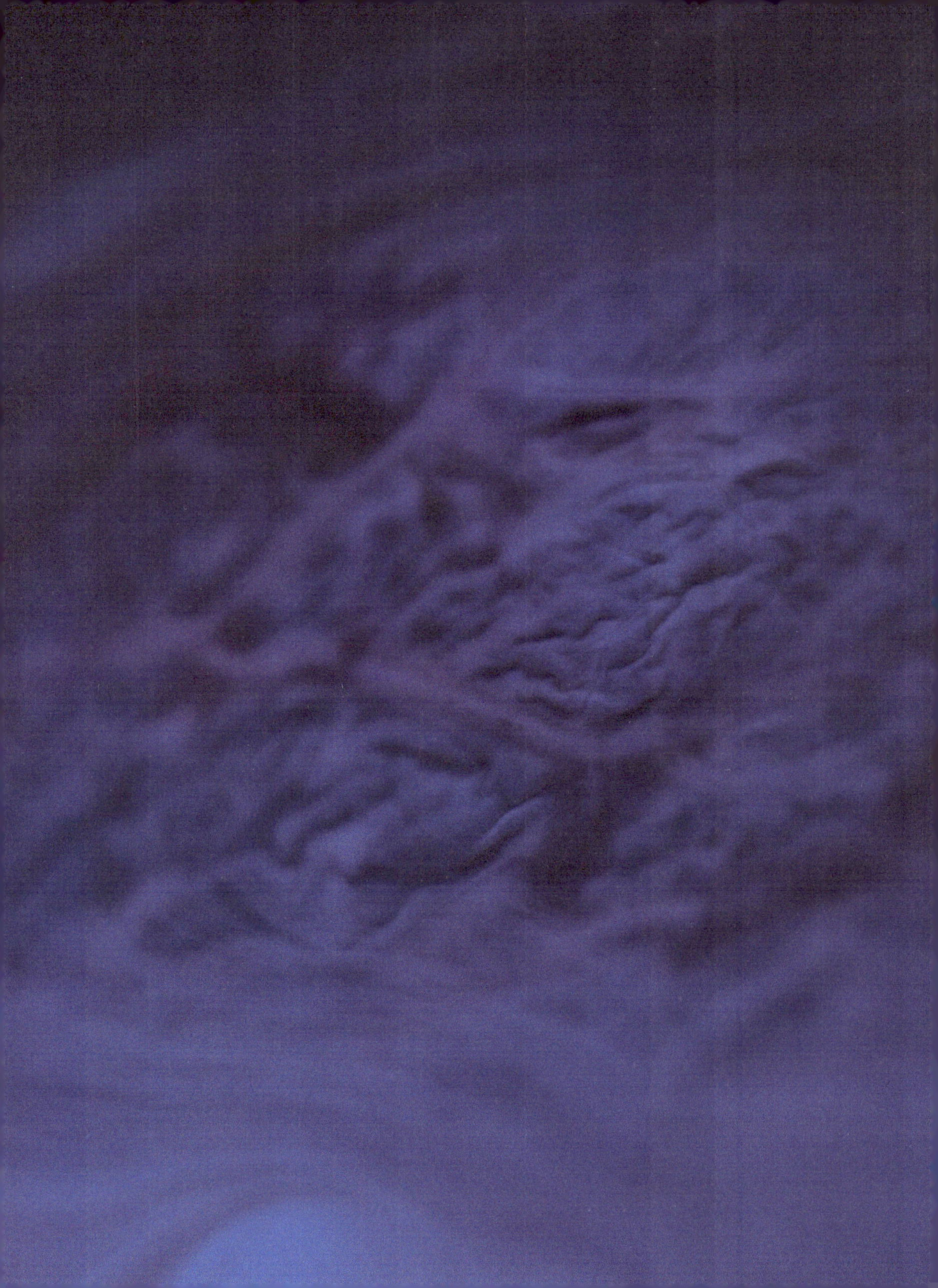

PREFACE TO THE ENGLISH TRANSLATION

We wrote this book a year ago in our mother tongue, German. In order to make our research and findings accessible to a wider audience, we have decided to translate "Plazenta Power" into English. However, this is purely a translation. It is not an adaptation for English-speaking or other countries, which means that we refer to German laws and regulations. Please note that the statements in this book may not be applicable, valid or legal in another country or state. We therefore ask you to undertake your own research on those topics independently.

Furthermore, the ideas and thoughts shared in this book might be influenced by our German culture. We ask for your understanding if we do not adequately reflect your customs, rules or culture. It is not our intention to judge or offend anyone in any way.

We are fascinated by all different kinds of placentas, no matter who gave birth to them!

Enjoy entering the placenta universe!

Sophia Johnson and Jana Pastuschek,
Weimar and Jena, June 2024

FOREWORD

An entire book just about the placenta? When the placenta simply "appears" after the birth? No, it is not simply that and the afterbirth is not just the "birth after birth". After the dramatic stretching of the vagina by the child, it allows the woman a further, much gentler stretching and soft birth - as a kind of reconciliation after the birth of the child; a soft, warm conclusion to this so formative birthday of her child.

The modern technical term "placenta" (Latin: cake) has replaced the long-used term "afterbirth". And that's a good thing. In common parlance, the placenta has long been called a mother´s cake and sometimes also a child's cake. These terms do far more justice to the organ. After all, it has nourished the child since its conception, allowing it to grow and thrive. No placenta, no child! Because without all these vital substances that the placenta produces and transports to the child via the umbilical cord, the growth of a child in the womb would not be possible. The placenta is also responsible for removing the baby's metabolic products - an all-round talent that offers a 24-hour service to the unborn child. The Mexican term "companion" or the term "other half", which is commonly used in Latvia, is therefore far more appropriate.

The placenta provides reliable care for the child, parents can trust it to a great extent and so they should also look at it after the birth and thank it for its perfect care. This was the baby's cradle during pregnancy: soft, red-blue-purple in color and covered with a delicate silk canopy (the egg membranes). I always said: Look, your child was wrapped in velvet and silk, soft and warm, take this as a model. Covered that way your child can continue to grow well "outside".

As you can read in this book, the placenta not only nourished the child in the womb, it is also a powerful healing agent for mother and child after birth. It is reassuring that there have always been parents who - presumably through conversations with midwives or like-minded people - give a lot of thought to what should happen to the organ after birth. Some bury it more or less secretly very deep in their own garden - others invite people to a ritual at the christening and plant a tree together with family and friends to match the shape of the placenta or the child's name, such as an apple tree of the same name for the boy Jonathan. Others prepare a homeopathic medicine themselves, some have it professionally made, others eat a piece raw - read about the healing power of the placenta in this book and then understand that there really is power in it!

So, this piece of "human flesh" is actually more important after the birth of the child than you might think. The two experts Sophia Johnson and Jana Pastuschek have succeeded in writing a book with a refreshing yet factual vocabulary that opens up scientifically confirmed new horizons for the placenta - the gory chunk of power after the birth of a child.

I hope that the book will become specialist literature for midwives and obstetrics, and that it will be an exciting read for parents-to-be, enabling them to make well-informed decisions about what they consider to be right for them with regard to the placenta after birth.

Ingeborg Stadelmann, June 2023

INTRODUCTION TO OUR PLACENTA UNIVERSE

"Hello Sophia, who's looking after your children tonight? I've just had a call from the delivery room: The midwives are currently looking after a woman giving birth to her second child, the cervix is fully dilated. It may well be that the placenta will be born in an hour or two. Could you come to the lab?"

This is roughly what a typical call from my colleague and now friend Jana Pastuschek sounds like. Together we have spent the odd night or two at the Placenta Laboratory at Jena University Hospital taking samples from newborn placentas. While the mother's attention is naturally focused on the newborn after birth, Jana and I find it incredibly exciting to devote ourselves to the "miracle organ of pregnancy", the placenta.

But that wasn't always the case ...

During my medical studies, the placenta was only mentioned as a side issue in the lectures on gynecology. It was only after the birth of my daughter that my husband surprised me by asking me whether he should make my placenta into capsules, as this would supposedly support healing in the postpartum period. He is half American and had already heard about the trend in the USA. However, I didn't know anything about it until then and rejected his suggestion. But my interest was piqued, so a few months later I knocked on the door of the placenta laboratory in Jena: "Have you ever heard of placenta as a remedy?" And so, my scientific work on this topic began.

All beginnings are dusty, because it is well known that exciting experiments are preceded by literature research. I spent a lot of time in libraries and sometimes had more than seventy-year-old, porous, typewritten pages of doctoral theses on placenta as a remedy in my hands. The further my research took me, the clearer it became to me: placenta is known to be an effective remedy in the various integrative medical systems such as homeopathy, anthroposophical medicine and traditional Chinese medicine.

I was then faced with the challenge of combining knowledge about the traditional use of the placenta with the modern fundamentals of research in obstetrics. Placenta as a remedy has not yet arrived in today's scientific world. There are only a few researchers worldwide who are working intensively on this topic, and one of them doesn't live in Las Vegas or Buffalo, but just around the corner: Jana Pastuschek.

"... I must have looked quite funny when Sophia knocked on the door of the laboratory and asked openly whether we had ever heard of the placenta as a remedy. I had been a research assistant at the placenta lab for five years at that point. The laboratory had even been in existence for decades. And yet neither I nor any of my colleagues had ever heard of it. Exciting, I thought, formidable topic, charismatic woman, coffee cup just full – so let's hear all the ideas floating around in the air and space.

At the time, there was too little (current) literature and studies for a theoretical doctoral thesis on the subject. And in my opinion, you can only research a placenta if you have held it in your own hands and felt its strength and power. As a biologist, I know that research is often laborious and time-consuming and that funding for it is virtually non-existent or has to be acquired at great expense with expertise in the respective field. Experiments and studies have to be planned within a feasible framework. Until sufficiently valid results are obtained, it is often a frustrating path that can be accompanied by a number of setbacks.

None of this deterred Sophia. We asked each other questions, planned experiments, looked for scientific supporters and cooperation partners, wrote an ethics application, started a crowdfunding campaign, raised more money than we had hoped for, educated midwives, asked expectant mothers to donate their placenta and got started: no matter what time of day, whether at the weekend or on a public holiday. We were delighted with every call and gratefully accepted the placentas donated to us. These, just like their babies, are not only born between 8 a.m. and 4 p.m., but of course around the clock. And so, this one afternoon of getting to know each other has turned into many hours, days and nights, weeks and months and now even more than eight years of joint research and friendship. What gives us strength to this day and often keeps us euphoric is our fascination with the miracle of the placenta: holding the source of human life in our hands, warm and fresh, and occasionally being able to listen to the child's first life-affirming cries at the same time."

Every placenta is unique. The development of this organ began around 140 million years ago because it gave newborns a better chance of survival. A relatively large placenta with a connection to the uterus, which supplies food and oxygen and removes metabolic products, enabled mammals to allow the unborn child to mature longer in the protected womb. A lot has happened since the development of the "primordial placenta", and it is now one of the organs with the greatest evolutionary diversity among animal species. For example, mice naturally have mouse placentas, elephants naturally have elephant placentas and humans have a human placenta.

Animal experiments cannot always be avoided in research. However, if we want to know something about human pregnancy, we can do so almost exclusively with human placentas. With a theoretical availability of almost 400 tons of placental tissue per year in Germany alone, this should not be a problem. (For those interested in numbers: In 2022, there were 739,000 newborns, multiplied by 500 grams of average placental weight, that's 369,500 kilograms of placental tissue.) So, without using or killing animals for our research, we can learn a lot about pregnancy and birth. As a nice karmic side effect, animal testing is automatically reduced.

But this is only possible thanks to the donations from the mothers. We authors would therefore like to take the opportunity to say thank you to the children and mothers for their gifts! We also appreciate the valuable cooperation between research and obstetrics and want to say thank you to the midwives who love their profession, even if external conditions are making this increasingly difficult.

For many birth attendants, the use of placenta is nothing new: Cornelia Enning wrote a book about the placenta ("Placenta – gift of life") back in 2003 – based on her experience as a midwife for many years. Of course, perspectives change according to the professional background. And so, we will take a look at this topic from a medical and a scientific perspective. It is important to remember that research sometimes develops at a rapid pace. Today we cannot prove scientifically how or if the placenta acts as a remedy, perhaps because we do not yet have the methods to do so. But maybe we will know more in fifty years' time. However, the Chinese physician Li Shizhen wrote as early as the 16th century that "(Placenta) is outstanding... Even the stupid will achieve effects when they use it." The experience gathered over years and centuries is not imaginary, but empirical. But there are also very loud, critical voices in the scientific debate about placenta as a remedy, and we would like to counter these with our clearly presented results. In our society, we would like to exclude as many risks as possible, and so the potential danger of placenta as a remedy is in the air. But conversely, could we also ask what risks arise for mother and child from not taking it? The experience of midwives shows: Women use their own placenta in the postpartum period – for example, a small piece pureed raw in a smoothie, or dried and processed into capsules or homeopathic medicine – and benefit from it, regardless of how significant the data is.

Every woman can and may do what she wants with her own placenta: leave it in the clinic, eat it as Bolognese, donate it for placenta research, process it into homeopathic medicine or bury it with dignity. Apart from a few obvious social rules (for example, that you shouldn't bury the placenta in a public park and leave the umbilical cord sticking out), the mother can decide what happens to the placenta. And at this moment it is not just about benefits or risks, but also about the woman's right to make self-determined decisions that affect only her personally, her own body and the organ that has grown in her womb together with the child. Every woman experience pregnancy, birth and the puerperium individually – and sometimes there is also a story about the placenta. That is why we have also given mothers a voice in this book, who gratefully share their own experiences with the placenta with us.

Unfortunately, the bubble of science rarely lands on public ground. What is discussed in English-language scientific publications often does not reach the women who are really interested in it. Sometimes it takes decades for the results of research to be incorporated into clinical or medical practice. We would like to present what we have found out, discussed and thought through during our joint research work here in an abridged and comprehensible form so that interested women can use this knowledge and make an informed decision for themselves. But we have also explained a lot of information in detail for birth companions such as midwives, doulas or obstetricians – those who find it too specific in individual cases are welcome to leaf through it. However, our book should not be confused with a guide to placenta consumption or therapy, as we lack the clinical experience for this.

But: For the one or other interested father who wants to really spoil his wife in the postpartum period, there are of course step-by-step instructions for a fresh fruit smoothie with a small piece of placenta and other recipe ideas in the appendix. Cheers!

FIELD REPORT BY ANDREA

The result in advance: I would do it again. In retrospect you never know what really caused which effects. But after the birth of my first son, I probably had something like a "mild depressive phase". At least friends tried to make me aware of this possibility from time to time, although I thought that slight dips in mood and a rather frequent lack of motivation were nothing that could be described as "depressive". People also tend to sugarcoat or romanticize everything that happened in the past. If it hadn't been for the second birth, I would not have realized that everything can look completely different. Thanks to a friend who had taken a course on processing placenta and wanted me to benefit from her knowledge, I was able to experience ingesting my placenta this time. A few hours after the birth, my friend was at home instructing my husband on how to process the placenta. Cut into thin strips, the placenta is dried for many hours in the oven at a low temperature, while my husband went to the pharmacy in search of one hundred and forty gelatin capsules and I enjoyed a fresh piece of placenta in the form of a fruit smoothie for dinner. So, I can't say anything about the taste of the placenta. It was lost in the pureed wild berries. The fact is that my involution (the shrinking of the uterus after childbirth) progressed so quickly that the doctors were always amazed when they felt for the "upper edge of the uterus", and I had no problems at all with milk production.

In the meantime, my husband had found the gelatin capsules and processed the dried placenta strips into a fine powder, which was then painstakingly filled into the capsules. My friend explained to me that I should now take these capsules every day during the postpartum period and beyond. I was open to everything and just wanted to see what happened. I can't say for sure whether this was due to the much easier second birth and my joy about it or whether the placenta had an effect. In any case, I think it's worth mentioning that despite a chronic lack of sleep (only four hours at night and thirty minutes during the day for a long period of time), I was in an incredibly good mood, almost euphoric, also because, contrary to my expectations based on my experiences of the first birth, I was doing really well and was able to do enjoy my day. As far as milk production was concerned, I could actually observe a connection with the placenta intake. During the first weeks after birth, I took two capsules a day, but I quickly had to reduce this to one capsule daily as my milk production had increased rapidly. Looking back, I can't say for how long I actually took the capsules. In any case, they ran out at some point and I think it's a shame that I don't still have some in reserve or that the placenta is only so "small" that I couldn't conjure up more products from it, because, as I have already read in many places, they can be used in many different ways – not only for the mother, but also for the child.

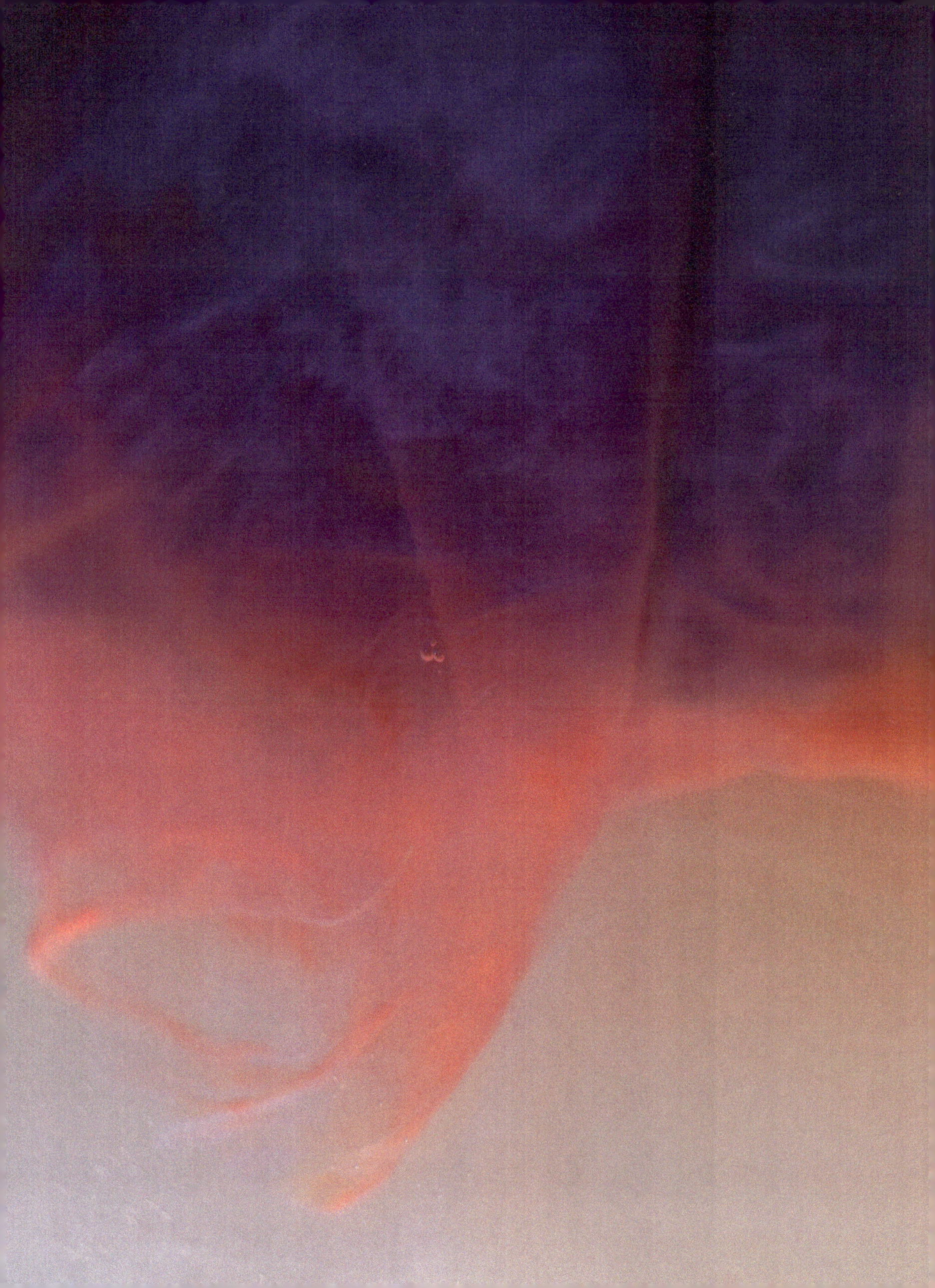

THE PLACENTA: MIRACLE ORGAN AND ALL-ROUNDER

We live in a world in which everything is in motion and flux, a constant change between polarities: sun - moon, day - night, mountain - valley, joy - sorrow ... and of course in the opposites of the very essential moments in life: birth and death. With the beginning of a new life, with the birth of a child, we also say goodbye to the organ that made pregnancy and birth possible in the first place.

Before we come to the question of whether the placenta is still important for the mother after birth, we would first like to look at its phylogenetic development (that is, its evolutionary history), formation and its tasks during pregnancy: the placenta as an immunological miracle organ, its microbiological peculiarity, the placenta as hormone factory, mouthpiece for environmental influences and female "all-rounder".

The phylogenetic origin of the placenta

The placenta is fascinating from an evolutionary perspective. The first forms of the placenta originated with the mammals (Mammalia) in the Cretaceous period around 140 million years ago. At this time, the dinosaurs were still populating the earth before they became extinct around 65 million years ago. In terms of phylogeny, the class of mammals branched out into the "Prototheria", the cloacal animals, which include the still living platypus and the echidna, as well as the "Theria". The Theria developed further into marsupials such as wombats, kangaroos and koalas on the one hand and into the higher mammals on the other.

Cloacal animals lay eggs, marsupials give birth to living offspring. Both already have a small, simple yolk-sac placenta, which in marsupials already serves to connect the embryo with the mother and provide nutrients. Gestation periods are still relatively short and the offspring are very small at birth, which makes months of further maturation and growth in the pouch necessary.

At 125 million years old, Eomaia ("mother of the dawn") is the oldest known fossil of higher mammals with a placenta. Higher mammals make up 94% of all mammal species living today and one of them is our human species. What they all have in common is a comparatively large and complex placenta connected to the uterus, which supplies the embryo or fetus with food and oxygen and removes waste products. The placenta enables a longer maturation and growth period for the offspring in the protected womb.

It used to be assumed that there was a hierarchical higher development of the species and also of the placenta. According to this idea, humans with their human placenta were at the top. Today we know that this is not the case. The human placenta is no more highly developed in evolutionary terms than the placenta of horses, cows or dogs. What is more important is that each type of placenta fulfills all functional requirements in order to produce a newborn that is optimally developed for the subsequent independent life of the respective species.

Placenta basics

The mature human placenta is deep red to purple, disc-shaped, weighs an average of 500 grams, is usually 2 to 3 centimeters thick and has a diameter of 15 to 20 centimeters. The placenta also includes the amniotic sac, medically known as the embryonic membrane. This consists of two parts, the chorion and the amnion, which surround the unborn child in the womb. The word "amnion" is derived from the Greek "amnos", meaning lamb. This is because when lambs are born in spring, some are still born with a closed amniotic sac, the so-called sheep's skin. "Chorion" (Greek: skin) is also interpreted as "the space maker" due to the many protrusions. At the beginning of pregnancy, the so-called villi form from the chorion, which, with their large surface area, enable an intensive exchange of nutrients. Towards the end of the third month, the villous covering on all sides recedes and the villi only remain in the disc-shaped area of the placenta.

The surface of the placenta facing the inner uterine wall is divided into many lobes, also known as cotyledons. These cotyledons are a functional sub-unit of the placenta. If you hold a newborn placenta in your hand, you can recognize it very clearly: The maternal side has a fissured surface. It had grown into the inside of the uterus until birth. The side facing the unborn child, on the other hand, is smooth and delicate, almost like silk. It is covered with a strong vascular pattern, often reminiscent of a tree of life. The umbilical cord, placenta and embryonic membranes are collectively referred to as the afterbirth.

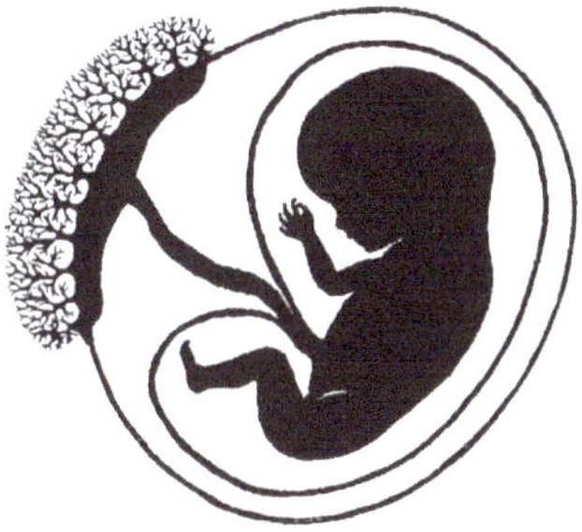

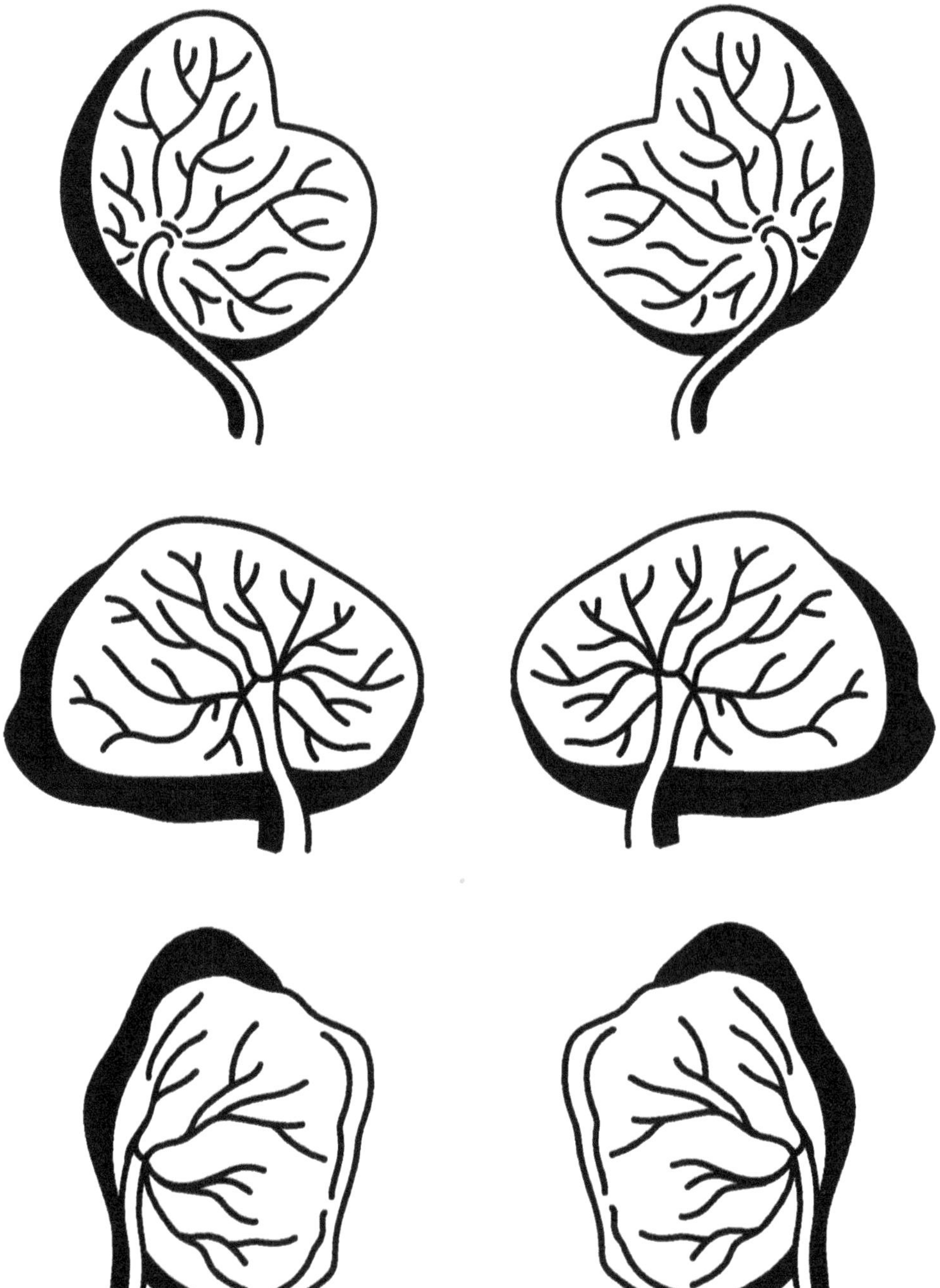

From the sphere to the disk

Fertilization must take place first, of course, before a placenta can develop. Two completely opposite germ cells - the round, female egg cell and the tiny, agile sperm cell - meet, merge and structure a completely new, individual life. Magic!

After fertilization, the germinal vesicle (also known as the blastocyst) forms, consisting of the embryoblast (the cell mass from which the embryo develops) and the trophoblast (from which parts of the placenta develop). During this stage of pregnancy, the fertilized egg is called "embryo". Parts of the placenta, the amniotic sac and the umbilical cord also develop from the cells of the embryoblast, which later becomes the child. They are therefore genetically from the same origin as the fetus.

During the implantation phase, the blastocyst attaches itself to the inner uterine lining (so called endometrium). It then grows completely into the endometrium, which is heavily supplied with blood. There the blastocyst nests and makes itself at home. The development of the placenta begins when the endometrium reacts to the presence of the embryo with metabolic activity. The placenta, which is initially spherical and envelops the embryo, changes its shape as it begins to be supplied with maternal blood. This happens towards the end of the first trimester of pregnancy. It then becomes disc shaped. A fetal side of the placenta is formed and a maternal side with the raised and fissured basic structure of the villous tree. The two sides form the whole of the placenta organ.

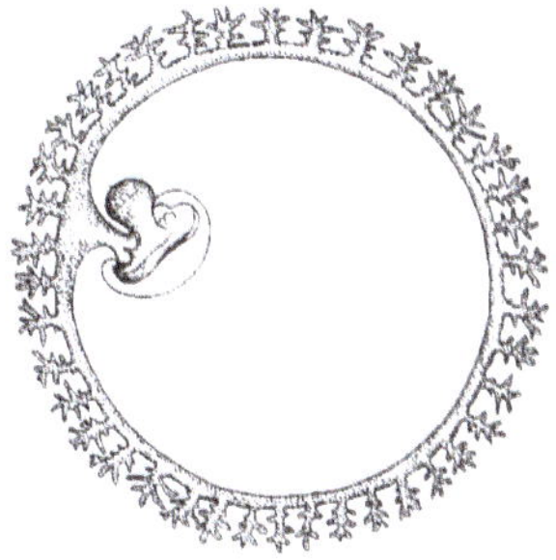

The placental metabolism

If you look at the structure of the placenta, the villous tree in particular stands out as an architectural masterpiece. Its numerous protrusions give it a much larger surface through which the metabolic dialog between mother and child takes place. These villi protrude into cavities in the endometrium, which are filled with maternal blood. Strictly speaking, the placenta is not yet supplied with "real" maternal blood in the first trimester of pregnancy, but only with a filtrate, a fluid still without blood cells. It is only towards the end of the first trimester that an influx of maternal blood with blood cells occurs. This close connection between maternal and fetal blood circulation enables an exchange of gases and metabolic products. However, there is no direct contact between maternal and fetal blood. This protective function of the placenta, also known as the placental barrier, regulates the transfer of substances from the mother to the child and vice versa.

One of the placenta's main tasks is to supply the unborn child with nutrients such as carbohydrates (in the form of glucose), amino acids (building blocks for proteins), fatty acids, trace elements and oxygen. For this purpose, the mother's organism, regulated by hormones, is brought into a metabolic state in favor of the child's energy requirements. This is to ensure that there are always sufficient nutrients and cell components in the mother's blood so that the unborn child is always adequately supplied.

No other organ is as efficient as the placenta – it continuously produces proteins and other important metabolic products and increases its output more and more as the pregnancy progresses.

When the placenta is working at full speed, it also produces a lot of heat. This aspect is of great importance, as maternal warmth naturally conveys much more to the unborn child than just temperature: security, relaxation and well-being.

The placenta has a high energy requirement and naturally also needs a lot of oxygen for the endless cell processes. This makes it even more understandable that pregnant women firstly need a good, healthy, energy-rich diet and secondly that they should take frequent deep breaths to ensure sufficient oxygen levels in the blood. So: fresh fruit and vegetables, nuts, nourishing soups and pregnancy yoga for the placenta!

Protection and defense – placental immunology

Mother and child are two independent living beings who share a home during pregnancy. But how can it be that "completely foreign" tissue with genetic information from another person is accepted without objection in the mother's body? This is a special situation for the immune system that would be inconceivable without the placenta. But the "immunology of reproduction" begins earlier: the uterus must protect itself from pathogens (it does this with good bacteria, as we discuss in the chapter *Hotly debated: Placenta and microbiome*), but at the same time it must not expel sperm with too much immune defense. The number of white blood cells (leukocytes) is already increasing at the end of the menstrual cycle, when a germinal vesicle might implant. Of these leukocytes, 70% are natural killer cells and are produced by the uterus. Once implantation has taken place, the immunological activity of the uterus increases and the number of immune cells also continues to rise.

The immunological challenge of pregnancy is to protect the uterus from infections on the one hand and to not reject the developing unborn child on the other. The placenta, in its function as an immunological balancing organ, enables mother and child to live together symbiotically. The balance of pro-inflammatory and anti-inflammatory hormones, immune cells and defense messengers released by the placenta is essential for the normal course of pregnancy. The exchange between the mother's and the child's immune system takes place via the blood, in a similar way to the metabolic processes. Maternal white blood cells and antibodies thus reach the unborn child and can protect it from infections while it is still in the womb.

The first trimester of pregnancy is characterized by a pro-inflammatory phase, as the implantation of the germinal vesicle is accompanied by an increase in inflammation-stimulating messenger substances in the endometrium. This can also be interpreted as an increased safety level, as the uterus must now carefully protect the implanting germ. After successful implantation, the pregnancy becomes somewhat calmer (immunologically speaking). The mother's organism is then in an anti-inflammatory state until this changes again at the time of birth.

The fine-tuning of the maternal immune system is incredibly complex and the subject of current research, especially when it comes to the development of diseases during pregnancy. The placenta is irreplaceable in its role as mediator. It regulates whether the immune system goes into a defensive posture or whether the child's development should be protected.

Hotly debated: Placenta and Microbiome

The immune system must be able to precisely recognize and distinguish whether it is confronted with friend or foe. The correct classification of foreign organisms, or pathogenic microorganisms in medical terms, therefore plays a major role. The fact that the placenta also harbors its own bacteria is the subject of lively debate in the scientific world. Therefore, we cannot avoid introducing the placental microbiome here. But we need to go into a little more detail.

The historical development of microbiology is extremely exciting, because until a few decades ago it was believed that bacteria were the cause of diseases. In Europe, since the middle of the 19th century, the idea was widespread that microorganisms are evil pathogens that make us suffer and sometimes even die. Protecting people from the invasion of these germs was the main medical goal and explains the euphoria surrounding the discovery of antibiotics. Research into the microbiome and its many facets in every conceivable niche of the body led to a paradigm shift.

What is the microbiome? It is exactly the two to three kilograms on the scales that we secretly think do not belong to us. Yet this entirety of microorganisms, i.e. bacteria, viruses and fungi and their genes, is vital for our survival. In every nook and cranny of the body, no matter how small, from the mouth to the intestines, the belly button to the vagina, a small, dynamic and interactive coexistence and interaction of microorganisms can be discovered. The specific microbiome is therefore a micro-ecosystem within a macro-ecosystem. We now know that not only does the gut have its own microbiome, but that all other organs such as the skin and the oral cavity also have one. What's more, your own microbiome is as unique as a fingerprint. It can influence an individual's predisposition to health or illness. Diet, but also stress, poor health status or the use of antibiotics can have an impact on our microbiome or throw it out of balance. This bacterial imprint of the mother's world is also transferred to the child via breast milk and intensive skin contact. Broken down to the essentials, it's something like this: Lifestyle and genetics determine the diversity of microorganisms and the more diverse the microbiome, the better.

A healthy person harbors a huge number of different microorganisms, which in their mass have more DNA than the person themself. There are more microorganisms in our body than our own body cells. Very few of them cause diseases or infections. What's more, our body cannot be healthy without this communicative coexistence. Imbalances can make life difficult for us and could lead to physical and mental illness.

The vaginal microbiome – sour makes you happy

Everyone, man and woman, knows that the vagina has a certain charm. However, not everyone knows that its microbiome is anything but charming but is generally acidic. When we write here about the pH value of the vaginal environment, we can say: acidic is healthy!

Around 9% of the total bacterial colonization of women is found in the vagina. More than 560 different species of bacteria live peacefully together here. Lactobacilli, also known as lactic acid bacteria, are the most prominent, with more than 120 species now known. By producing hydrogen peroxide and lactic acid, they lower the pH value of the vagina into the acidic range. Disease-causing germs then feel less at home. The healthy vaginal flora from puberty to the menopause is dominated by these small, rod-shaped microorganisms. If this lactobacilli dominance is lost, the pH value rises and disease-causing bacteria multiply, which can lead to vaginal inflammation. Itching is inevitable!

In the non-pregnant state, the composition of the vaginal flora is subject to age-related, cyclical, hormonal, ethnic and, of course, sexual influences. Different types of lactobacilli alternate in their dominance. During pregnancy, the vaginal microbiome is much more stable, albeit less species rich and variable. If, however, the balance determined by lactobacilli is disturbed, premature rupture of the membranes, premature birth, inflammation of the uterus or placenta and infection of the unborn child can occur as a result of an emerging vaginal infection.

Therefore: Lactic acid bacteria belong in the vagina! They are valuable protectors of pregnancy and women should not drive them out with excessive hygiene! From the point of view of the vaginal microbiome, you can understand why there is a trend in industrialized countries towards not washing. Because once the local bacterial flora has been removed by alkaline detergents, it takes a long time until a healthy and acidic balance is regained.

On everyone's lips: the placental microbiome

And you can take that literally: The composition of the microorganisms in the placenta most closely resembles those in our oral cavity. But this is still being debated in the scientific world. In a nutshell, the chronology is as follows: For the past hundred years, it was assumed that the unborn child would mature in a "germ-free", i.e. sterile, environment. According to this idea, the transmission of diseases only occurred through an infection of the mother during pregnancy or during birth. Today, we know that there are very specific clusters of microorganisms, depending on who or what is being examined: the unborn child, the placenta, the amniotic fluid or the newborn's first stool (medically known as meconium, in Germany known as "child's tar" because of its color).

In 2014 came the great scientific proclamation: the placenta has its own microbiome! As is always the case with changing the status quo, counter-publications were of course published immediately. Currently supporters and opponents of this theory are carrying out a heated debate about whether the placenta harbors its own microbiome or not. Perhaps contamination during sampling and analysis has led to an unsustainable hypothesis after all? In any case, we are excited to see what light future research results can shed on our current knowledge of the placental microbiome.

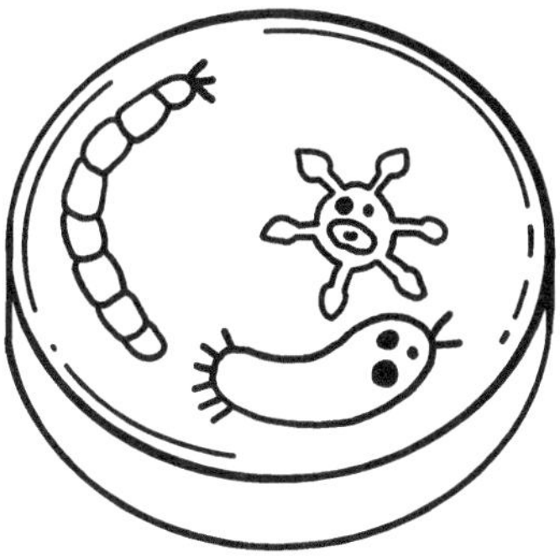

The placenta as a hormone factory

Hormones are the body's own messenger substances and they form their own very complex communication system. They not only regulate metabolism and the function of organs and glands, but also, for example, our mood or how we deal with relationships. There are many places in the human organism where hormones are produced. For example, the thyroid gland is known for its production of thyroid hormones, the pancreas for its production of insulin – and the hormonal activity of the gut is also attracting more and more medical attention. Information is sent from the gut to the brain via the gut-brain axis and thus regulates mental health, among other things. Conversely, the connection between the brain structures of hypothalamus and pituitary gland and the adrenal cortex regulates the body's reaction to stress. And the placenta, with its very own production of hormones, bursts into the middle of this sophisticated system of hormone production and activity. In terms of its creative power, the placenta is a marvel: it produces pregnancy-promoting, pregnancy-stabilizing and birth-inducing hormones at a sometimes exponential rate. The amount of hormones produced increases with the weight of the placenta. The only exception in this case is human chorionic gonadotropin (hCG), a hormone that is important in the early stages of pregnancy. The increase in hCG is also used in pregnancy tests. It can already be detected in early pregnancy and its concentration rises rapidly at the beginning, with the concentration doubling approximately every second day. During this time, the woman may also feel "somehow different". If the implantation of the fertilized egg was successful, hCG slowly decreases again from around the third month of pregnancy and the other hormones take over. This is often the time when the pregnant woman starts to feel better again.

Progesterone plays a major role in maintaining pregnancy. It safeguards and protects the pregnancy. The placenta produces progesterone at an exponential rate and the concentration of this hormone increases tenfold during pregnancy. It prepares the woman's breasts for breastfeeding and has a pain-relieving and antispasmodic effect. Progesterone also protects the uterus from premature activity; if the muscles of the uterus were to contract at the wrong time, premature labor could occur.

Also important for pregnancy are estrogens, the female hormones that ensure beautiful skin, full hair and a woman's special glow during pregnancy. They stimulate the growth of the uterus and mammary glands as well as blood flow to the uterus and placenta. Estrogens also promote the production of other hormones by the placenta.

Estrogens and progesterone belong to the group of steroid hormones. These are fat-soluble hormones that develop from the precursor, cholesterol.

Another important pregnancy hormone produced by the placenta is human placental lactogen. The root word "lacto" comes from the Latin word "lac" for milk. Lactogen means milk promoting. And this is also the most important property of placental lactogen: it promotes milk production and also ensures that there are always enough nutrients available in the mother's blood for the unborn child. In terms of nutrition, it could therefore also be described as the all-inclusive hormone. The task of these placental hormones is to secure and support the pregnancy and to meet all the needs of the unborn child.

There is another group of very important pregnancy hormones that differ slightly in their function from the previous ones: the neurohormones. These hormones have an effect on the central nervous system and are significantly involved in stress management. These neurohormones include, for example, CRH (corticotropin-releasing hormone) and ACTH (adrenocorticotropic hormone). These regulate the body's response to internal and external stress factors. CRH ensures that ACTH is released. ACTH ensures that cortisol is released. And cortisol can then develop its pain-relieving and anti-inflammatory effect in the body.

These stress hormones are of course extremely important during childbirth. There is hardly any situation in life in which such high CRH concentrations can be measured in the blood as during a natural birth. The placenta enables a relaxed birth through the production of neurohormones and the release of pain-relieving and anti-inflammatory substances.

And then there is another essential hormone without which childbirth would not be possible: oxytocin. This "love hormone", sometimes also described as the "hormone of love and happiness", is very important for the maternal bond with the child and also regulates complex social and emotional behavior. It also ensures that the uterus contracts quickly after birth to prevent excessive blood loss. When the newborn is nursed, oxytocin ensures the flow of milk. The mother can tell whether the baby is feeding properly when the uterus contracts at the same time as the baby sucks on the breast. In addition, the body's own oxytocin provides the magical and loving aura that surrounds mother and child after the birth.

After this short excursion into the inner workings of the placental hormone factory, we can summarize: The interplay of placental hormones is incredibly complex and very harmonious. They activate each other and interact in such a way that the hormone spiral slowly and continuously increases over the weeks of pregnancy. But what happens after the placenta is born?

The hypothesis of postnatal hormone withdrawal

While the placenta is performing all its tasks, working at full capacity and continuing to increase in productivity as the pregnancy progresses, all is well! Pregnancy is characterized by a completely crazy hormonal situation: in the mother's peripheral blood an enormous amount of progesterone, estrogen and cortisol is measurable, to which the body has become accustomed step by step over 280 days. However, the hormonal high comes to an abrupt end with the birth of the placenta. This "hormone withdrawal", including hormones affecting the brain, is seen as the cause of postnatal mood swings, which can manifest as baby blues and even postpartum depression.

Of course, this is not the case for all women, but on a hormonal level it is easy to explain and understand that a mother can become quite unbalanced after giving birth. Fortunately, the female hormone balance regulates itself again over time. How long this takes, however, depends entirely on the individual birth situation, breastfeeding and many external factors that can influence health in the postpartum period.

After this brief insight into pregnancy hormones – which really only scratches the surface of the secrets of the placenta – we can say that it is a typically female organ: it performs multitasking at the highest level. Without the placenta, there would be no pregnancy and no newborn. An international holiday should definitely be dedicated to it!

At a glance: important hormones produced by the placenta

Human chorionic gonadotropin (hCG)

- key hormone for the implantation of the embryo
- enables continuity of pregnancy
- consists of two chains (α and β) – the β chain is responsible for hormone-specific activity
- ensures the continuous production of estrogen and progesterone by the corpus luteum
- immobilizes the uterine muscles

Progesterone

- belongs to the progestogens, i.e. the pregnancy-promoting hormones (Latin: gestare – to carry)
- most important pregnancy hormone
- produced exponentially by the placenta from the 6th week of pregnancy on with a tenfold concentration increase up to the 3rd trimester (production rate: 300 milligrams per day shortly before the delivery date)
- secures and protects pregnancy
- prevents the uterus from contracting
- prepares the mammary glands for breastfeeding
- has analgesic and antispasmodic properties

Estrogens

- the most common estrogens are estrone, estradiol and estriol
- after the 7th week of pregnancy, more than 50% of the estrogens in the mother's blood are produced by the placenta
- they prepare the mammary glands for breastfeeding
- they promote the growth of the uterus and uterine muscles and the flow of blood through the uterus and placenta
- they stimulate prostaglandin production by the endometrium

Human placental lactogen (hPL)

- has a similar structure to prolactin
- has a strong lactation-promoting effect
- extremely high secretion rate of 1 to 3 grams per day around the time of delivery
- influences the mother's metabolism (fat breakdown, counteracts insulin), thereby increasing the supply of nutrients for the unborn child and placenta, protects against low blood sugar (hypoglycemia)

Corticotropin-releasing hormone (CRH)

- is an essential neurohormone, similar to hypothalamic CRH
- regulates the body's response to stress
- produced exponentially by the placenta during pregnancy, highest concentration in the blood during vaginal birth
- stimulates prostaglandin and oxytocin release and stimulates estrogen synthesis
- causes the release of ACTH: the placental response to birth stress
- influences the contraction of the uterine muscles

Adrenocorticotropic hormone (ACTH)

- ACTH produced by the placenta has the same structure as ACTH produced by the pituitary gland in the brain
- supports placental steroid hormone synthesis
- promotes increased cortisol production and release by the adrenal glands
- endogenous cortisol acts on the metabolic system (provides energy by breaking down fats, increases blood sugar levels) and on the immune system (suppresses the immune system's response, has an anti-inflammatory effect)

Oxytocin (here we are referring to the body's own oxytocin, not the synthetically produced hormone)

- potent and specific hormone that stimulates birth and triggers the contraction of the uterine muscles
- initiates and promotes milk flow (triggered by suckling)
- 3 to 4-fold increase in synthesis at the time of birth
- key hormone for complex emotional and social behavior (bonding, maternal behavior, social recognition)
- was long regarded as the "hormone of love and happiness"

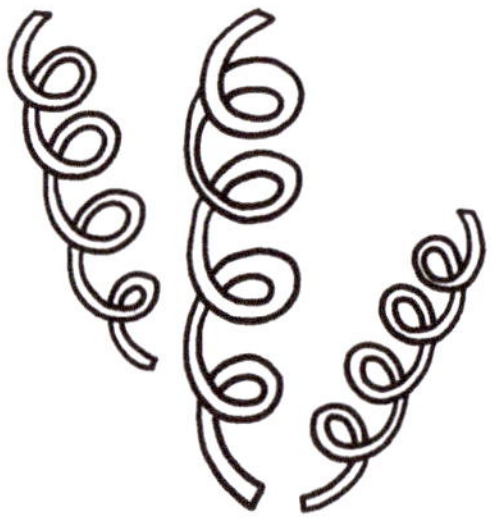

Overview of hormones produced by the placenta

(Table modified from Reis und Petraglia 2001)

Neuropeptides	Pituarity-like Hormones	Steroid Hormones	Monoamines and Adrenal-like Peptides
CRH	ACTH	Progesterone	Epinephrine
TRH	TSH	Estradiol	Norepinephrine
GnRH	GH	Estrone	Dopamine
Melatonin	PL	Estriol	Serotonin
Cholecystokinin	CG	2-Methoxy-estradiol	Adrenomedullin
Met-enkephalin	LH	Allopregnanolone	
Dynorphin	FSH	Pregnenolone	
Neurotensin	β-Endorphin	5α-Dihydropro-gesterone	
VIP	Prolactin		
Galanin	Oxytocin		
Somatostatin	Leptin		
CGRP	Activin		
Neuropeptide Y	Follistatin		
Substance P	Inhibin		
Enothelin			
ANP			
Renin			
Angiotensin			
Urocortin			

The birth of the placenta

The baby is here – birth is over! Or not quite yet?

For midwives and obstetricians, there is one more important moment after delivery: the birth of the placenta. Only when the placenta has been born the birth is complete and the parents are congratulated on their newborn!

However, we know from anecdotes told by mothers that the afterbirth was not always given any significance. Some women were surprised by the birth of the placenta after the baby was born because they didn't know about it. In modern hospitals it was not customary to show the afterbirth to the mother after delivery. The obstetricians were only interested in whether the placenta was completely delivered and therefore no further complications were to be expected. Then the placenta ended up in the hospital waste bin.

This has changed over the years. Today, there are many different ways of handling the placenta, depending on the place of birth, type of birth and individual care. Some mothers prefer a so-called "lotus birth", in which the umbilical cord is not cut after the birth, but the baby remains connected to the placenta via the umbilical cord. Only when the umbilical cord has dried and detaches from the baby's navel are newborn and afterbirth separated. More often, the umbilical cord is cut immediately after the baby has been delivered – for practical and hygienic reasons, among others: Woman can lay the newborn on her bare chest to cuddle without the connection to the placenta being "in the way". The situation is completely different with a caesarean section. It is often not possible for the mother to catch a glimpse of the placenta, as she cannot see the birth through a sterile drape in the operating room. But regardless of whether the baby is born naturally or by caesarean section, every placenta is thoroughly examined by midwives and obstetricians after the birth.

At a glimpse: Pulsation of the umbilical cord

When the child is born, there is still a connection to the placenta via the umbilical cord. This means that the child and placenta still have a common blood circulation. You can think of the placenta as a solid sponge that is filled with a lot of blood. As long as the umbilical cord is still pulsating, fetal blood flows from the placenta to the newborn through the umbilical cord vessels. This means that the proportion of blood volume in the newborn's circulation increases with the length of time that passes before the connection between the newborn and placenta is severed by the umbilical cord.

Anyone who has ever been lucky enough to hold a placenta in their hand, perhaps even their own, can certainly confirm that it is something very natural and fascinating.

When the placenta is freshly born, it is warm and soft. A little slippery, not very bloody. It hardly smells at all, and if it does, it's a slight mineral smell, like that of salt water or liquid iron. Very subtle. It lies there, broad and heavy. It is a selfless organ, made to give. Always on the child's side, it organizes everything that belongs to a good life: warmth, protection and cocooning, nourishment, fresh air in the form of oxygen and, of course, mediation and communication with the outside world. It absorbs everything that the child no longer needs, transports away, digests, cleanses, detoxifies, protects and remains in the background. It knows the wishes of the unborn child even before they can be formulated.

Sometimes the placenta can already show signs of age at birth. In this case its vessels are calcified. This can feel like sand or crumbs between the fingers, perhaps also lumps or nodules. Here and there the placenta may also have had small areas with insufficient blood circulation that are no longer functional and have been transformed into scar tissue. This shows how worn out the placenta is and how many weeks it has already had been working 24/7. The placenta is not made for a long life. With the birth of the child, the organ has fulfilled its task and can say goodbye – or not quite yet?

Pregnancy accomplished

Placenta birth

The detachment of the placenta usually begins after the birth of the baby. It usually takes a few strong postpartum contractions and the placenta is completely detached from the inner wall of the uterus. The detached placenta is expelled from the uterus into the birth canal – a blood loss of 200 to 400 milliliters and a duration of 10 to 30 minutes until the placenta is delivered is normal. In a squatting position, the placenta can also be delivered just two to three minutes after the baby is born; blood loss is often minimal as the uterus can contract again quickly.

Examination of the newborn placenta

The examination for completeness of the placenta after birth is usually carried out by midwives and obstetricians. The apparent changes to the placenta are examined. The diameter and weight of the placenta are also documented. The maternal side and the baby's side, including the membranes, are then inspected.

The focus here is on the completeness of the placenta: Is it completely delivered or is a piece missing? (This would mean that placental remnants would have to be recovered by scraping out the uterus in the operating room, otherwise there is a risk of secondary bleeding or infection.) Are there perhaps also secondary placentas, i.e. small round appendages to the main placenta? The membranes are also examined; these should be clear.

A clouding of the membranes can be an indication of an infection; greenish membranes are found after birth stress of the newborn, namely when meconium has passed during birth and the amniotic fluid has turned green.

The birth of the placenta ends the birth phase of the newborn. Only then is the mother congratulated.

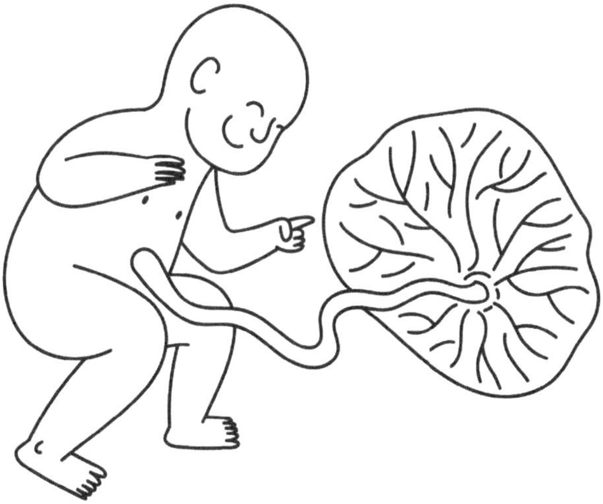

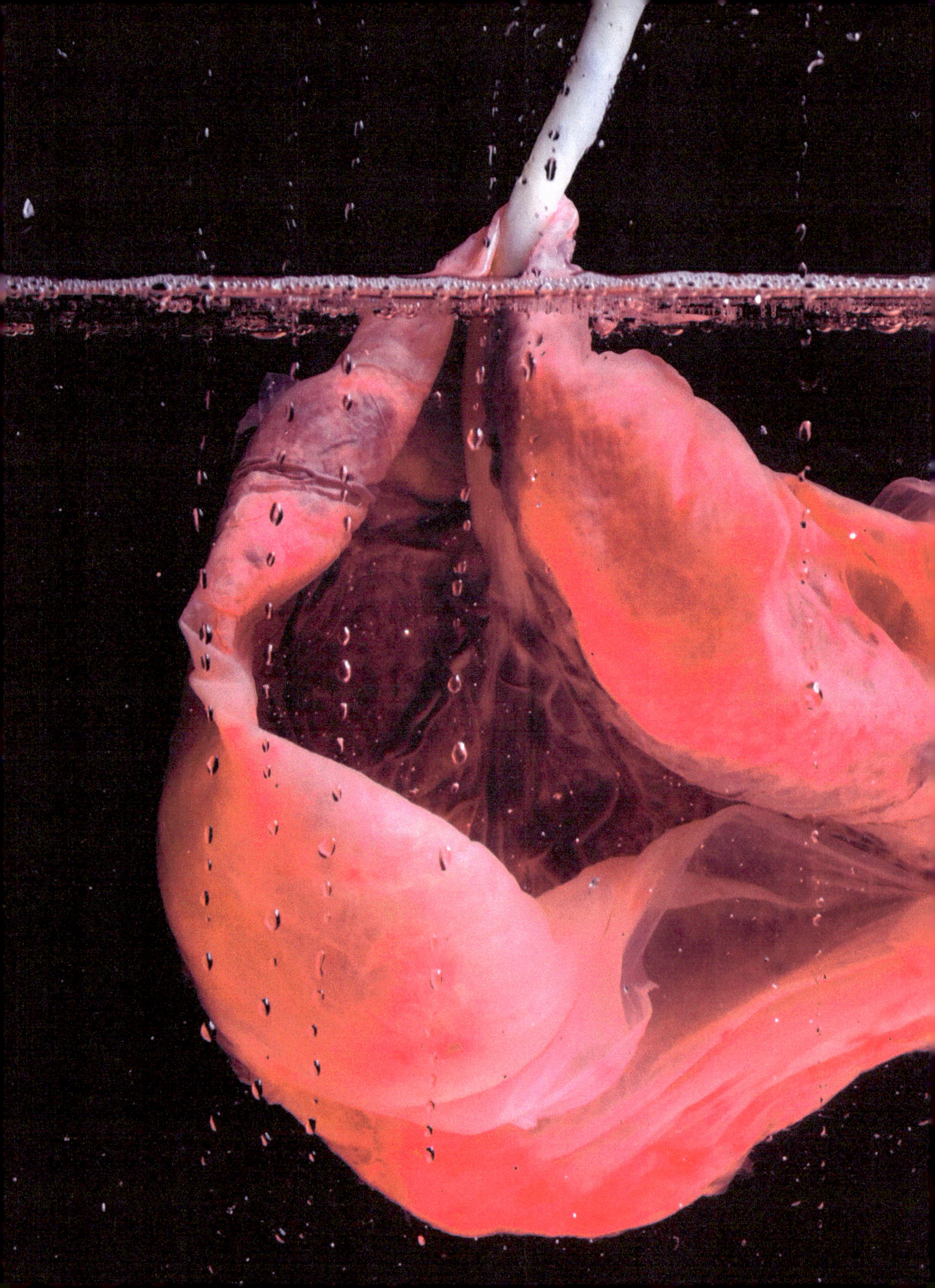

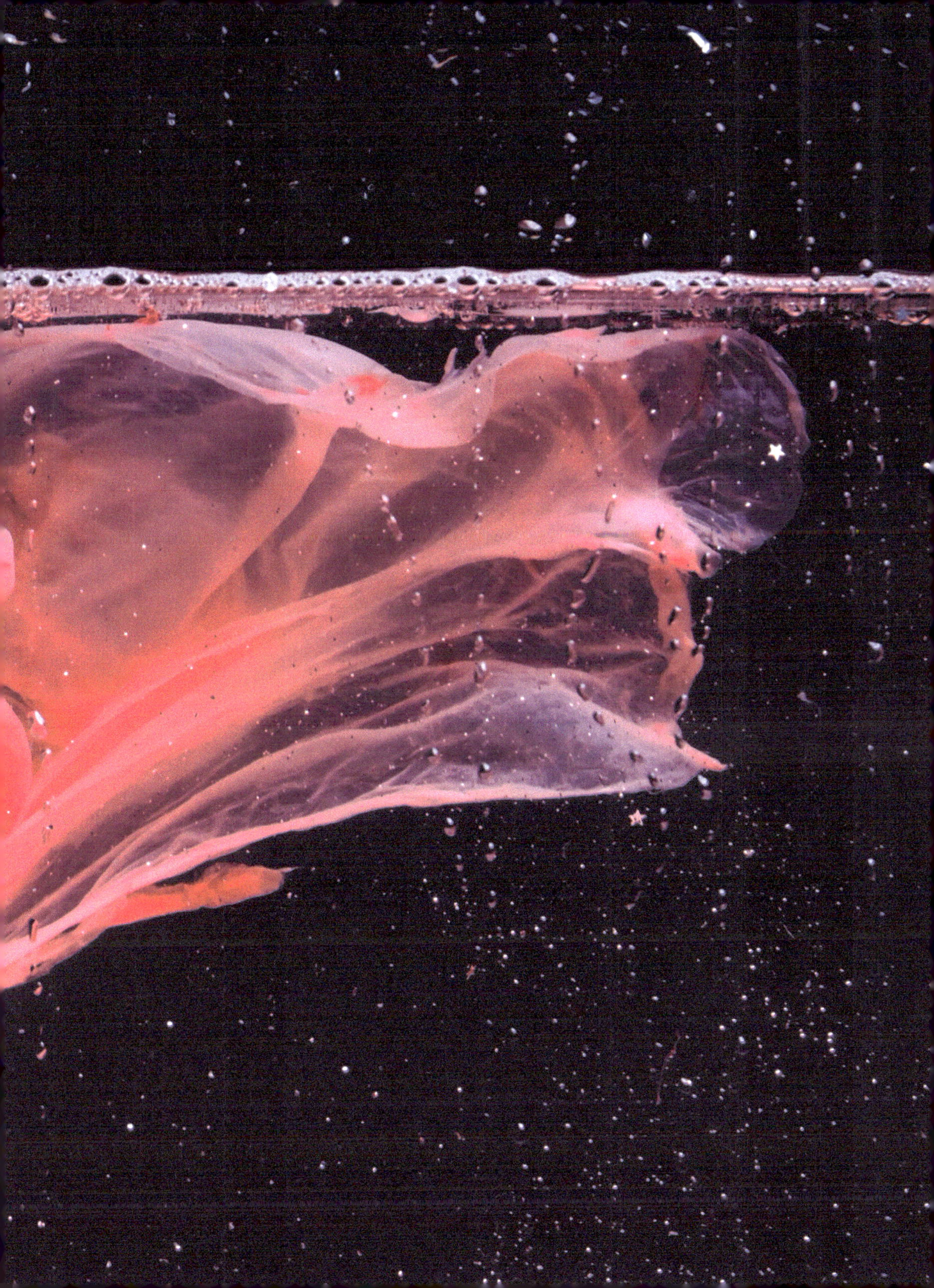

THE RITUAL USE OF THE PLACENTA

With so much attention given to the birth of a child, the small moment of saying goodbye to the placenta is often overlooked. In this day and age, this organ, which is an important and essential part of pregnancy, is rarely said goodbye to. However, this has not always been the case. There are rites and customs throughout the ages and cultures, all of which are variations of placenta funerals and accord great respect and appreciation to this miraculous organ. What all rituals have in common is that they aim to ensure the well-being and health of the child by giving the placenta a proper burial. It used to be said that if the placenta was safe, so was the child.

In addition, the placenta has always been closely associated with a woman's fertility. Global customs and rites were typically based on the four elements – fire, water, air and earth. The placenta was most frequently given to the earth, buried in leaves, cloth or pots, with or without other protective or fate-guiding gifts, in secret or in connection with small celebrations. The most common burial is under trees, often close to the house, or directly next to or in the house.

In the *Ben Cao Gang Mu* – a Chinese compendium of traditional medicines by the 16th century physician Li Shizhen – it is stated: "All placentas should be buried at a propitious place where they benefit from the virtue of heaven and the virtue of the moon."

There is a similar tradition from the early modern period in western culture: in southern Germany, the placenta should be buried "where neither the sun nor the moon shines". Although this is in direct contrast to the Chinese burial site, it is also meaningfully aligned with the stars. Perhaps the German indication was merely of a practical nature: People wanted to make sure that the afterbirth was not dug up and eaten by animals – as this would have had bad consequences for the newborn according to the beliefs of that time.

The discovery of so-called placenta pots has opened up a very special archaeological niche: In the rural areas of Baden-Württemberg, more precisely in Bönnigheim and the surrounding area, excavations have brought to light a special form of afterbirth burial from the past. The afterbirths were buried in the protected cellar of the house for several centuries, at least from the 17th to the 19th century. Clay pots specially designed for burial were used for this purpose, sealed with lids and sometimes turned upside down. Analyses of organic residues in the pots showed a high proportion of cholesterol (as a building material for hormones) and estradiol, which very probably originated from human placental tissue. Perhaps the placenta pots were also placed in the cellar with the household spirits to appease them by making an offering and thus giving them the most valuable thing that had come into the world together with the child. The pots were often painted with symbols and were probably included in ritual acts such as defensive or healing spells. The *Dictionary of German Superstition states* that the placenta was often attributed supernatural and particularly healing powers.

Many other ethnic groups also believe that the placenta is a spiritual being with a connection to the child. For example, some groups see the placenta or umbilical cord as the seat of the outer soul of the human being. This is also expressed in the many names that exist for the placenta, such as twin, unborn half, soul brother, the praised one, the robe of the immortal or Buddha's outer vestment.

In the Old Testament, 1 Samuel (24:29), we find the following wording from Abigail addressed to David: "And if a man has set out to persecute you and to seek your soul, then the soul of my territory shall remain bound up in the bundle of life with the Lord your God; but the souls of your enemies he will hurl out as from the bay of a sling." According to anthropologists James Frazer and Margaret A. Murray, the "bundle of life" refers to the placenta.

Even in Ancient Egypt, the placenta was seen as the seat of a person's outer soul. The placenta of a pharaoh was mummified and used as an insignia of power, a venerable and extremely valuable object. Together with the pharaoh himself, the well-being of the entire people depended on this outer soul of the pharaoh. When the pharaoh died, the "opener of the royal placenta" (a particularly high-ranking official in Ancient Egypt) symbolically opened the bundle so that both souls could reunite in divinity.

The placenta and its different (historical) names around the world	
German-speaking countries	Mutterkuchen – mother´s cake
English-speaking countries	after birth
French-speaking countries	arriere-faix, deliver, deliverance (salvation, rescue)
Polynesia (Tahiti)	pufenua (core of the earth) – nourishing character, strong connection to mother earth
New Zealand (Maori)	whenua (land that a tribal group uses together)
Graeko-Walachen	little house of the child
Southeast Asia (Hmong)	child's jacket (child's first and best clothing)
Southern Germany	"rot Wammesch", red doublet
Cameroon (Bayangam)	lin (seat or armchair of the child)
Uganda (Baganda)	twin of the child
Latvia	the other half
Mexico (Yucatan)	el compañero (companion of the child)
Mafa (North Cameroon)	little sister
Ancient Egypt	seat of the outer soul, bundle of life

(summarized according to Tchuitcheu 2010)

The worship and ritual use of the placenta was not only described in Egyptian and Arabic culture, but also across the borders of North Africa and into the regions south of the Sahara. There are many sources about placenta customs in Africa, ranging from the distant past to the 20th century.

Cross-cultural similarities can be found in the spiritual interpretation of the afterbirth: placenta and umbilical cord represent a connection between the parallel, invisible, divine ancestral world and this world; the points of contact between these two worlds are birth and death.

The fact that the placenta moves between sun and moon, heaven and earth, life and death, gives it this special, perhaps superstitious, but definitely magical meaning. It is therefore understandable that the placenta was treated with the greatest respect, whether used for ritual or therapeutic purposes.

FIELD REPORT BY LAURA

Even while I was working as a midwife, I noticed that women who took the placenta after the birth of their child felt positive effects. After the birth of my first child, I finally had the opportunity to try placenta myself and experience the effects on my own body.

My pregnancy and birth were without complications and my son was born relaxed and stress-free at home. After the birth, I ingested a piece of raw placenta about 2 centimeters in size and drank a placenta smoothie every day for the next three days. My milk came in particularly quickly, on the second day after the birth. My son had breast milk stools on the third day and was back to his birth weight by the fourth day. My uterus also regressed quickly. After nine days, it was no longer palpable from the outside.

I dried and pulverized the rest of the placenta and processed the powder into capsules. These capsules are still my little "instant helpers" today. As soon as I notice that I need more milk, for example due to my son's growth spurt or because I am experiencing more stress in my everyday life, I take two capsules once or twice a day. I usually notice in the same night that my milk production increases, and I can also cope better with the additional stress by taking placenta capsules.

After this experience as a midwife and mother, I can confirm that taking the placenta has a positive effect. Amongst other things on milk production, postnatal recovery and the ability to cope better with stressful situations.

HISTORY AND CURIOSITIES

Today, the placenta is often viewed solely as a pregnancy organ that must function properly to ensure the healthy development of the unborn child. Apart from this, there is another way of looking at the role of the placenta: the placenta as a healing agent after birth. However, this knowledge is nowadays not very popular and cannot be found in the relevant textbooks on obstetrics, but only - if at all - in references from traditional midwifery. This is demonstrated by midwife Cornelia Enning in her book *Heilmittel aus Plazenta*.

There are many different reports, anecdotes and traditions about the use of human placenta as a remedy around the world. In Argentina, for example, native ethnic groups use the powder from the dried umbilical cord to treat sick children. The Kol ethnic group in central India administer placenta as a remedy to improve fertility. The benefits are also known in other parts of Asia: A Chinese scientist who visited our placenta lab in Jena for a research exchange told us that, as a child, he was given a soup cooked with a small piece of his dried placenta and umbilical cord because he was so small and weak ... The list could go on and on.

From the Pharmacopoeia by Landamman

The use of placenta as a remedy - at least in German-speaking countries - can be traced back not only to traditional midwifery knowledge, but also to traditions from medical literature. In the pharmacies of the 18th century, dried placenta was available as a remedy alongside many other medicines of the time. There are various historical sources that document this. In the *Württemberger Pharmakopöe*, a pharmacopoeia from 1741, it is described that dried human placenta was administered as a powder for "difficult births". According to this source, the placenta was first washed in wine and then dried. This was a simple method of disinfection at the time, as wine was more sterile than water, which was often contaminated with germs.

Another historic written, the *Biblischer Medicus* from 1743, contains a similar statement: "The afterbirth, Secundina humana, dried up, has a special power to drive the birth and afterbirth." Women were probably given a spoonful of this powder during childbirth or when the afterbirth was delayed. As hormones such as oxytocin can be detected in dried placental tissue (we will go into this in more detail in the chapter *What´s in it?*), the powder could be described as an "18th-century oxytocin drip". (A little trip back in time: In modern obstetrics, synthetically produced oxytocin was used for many years as a nasal spray, as hormones administered via the oral and nasal mucous membranes are fast acting).

45. Für die Fallendsucht; sagt er mier den 8. augusti 1659.

Nimb das bürdeli [Nachgeburt] von einer Frauwen, so das erst kind gebirt vnd ein Sohn ist, doch daß es nit zuo boden gfallen, wesch solches mit win vnd ders am schaten auff dem offen, stoß es zuo bulffer; gib einem mentschen ein quintli des bulffers in lindenblust oder schlüßelblümli in [ein] im krebs, du solt aber wüßen, daß du im ersten tag, wan der mon im kreps ist, dan am andern tag im kreps gib ihm dis bulffer, in 4 wuchen gib ihms wider also im kreps mit purgieren vnd bulffer, vnd dan wider das drite mal wie zuo vor, so hilffts; die purgatz soll sein von Senet; min Recept ist gutt, von Senet mit Rosindli vnd Enis.

Reference from the historic Pharmacopoeia by Michael Schorno von Schwyz, Swiss Archive for Folklore: Reference for the traditional use of pulverized placenta to prevent seizures.

From the Pharmacopoeia by Landamman Michael Schorno from Schwyz

Outside of obstetrics, dried placenta was also used for therapeutic purposes in the 17th century. This can be found in the pharmacopoeia of the Landammann Michael Schorno of Schwyz (Landamann is the historical term for the head of the government of a Swiss rural municipality). He describes the use of placenta in the treatment of "falling sickness", or epilepsy. Dried placenta powder was mixed with aniseed and raisins and taken at monthly intervals. It is interesting to note that there are also references to the administration of placenta for epilepsy in the literature of Chinese and anthroposophical medicine.

What all the above-described treatment methods have in common is that they used the placenta as an organ that contains a special mix of hormones in its tissue. For a significant period within the 19th century, a great deal of experimentation was carried out to explore organ therapy (and the effects hormones, extracted from animal organs, may have). At that time, pharmacology was in its beginnings, and it was not yet possible to produce hormones artificially, so animal hormone glands were mainly used. The use of organs as therapeutics is called "opotherapy".

Various experiments were carried out in France, for example with fluids squeezed from animal testicles. The physiologist and neurologist Charles-Édouard Brown-Séquard injected himself with these organ extracts and, according to his own account, felt thirty years younger afterwards. As a result, the medical fraternity experienced an "organ hype" and the desire for eternal youth became the subject of research. The case of a patient who suffered from puffy and swollen skin (medically referred to as myxedema) due to hypothyroidism was sensationally celebrated. After she was treated with an extract of a sheep's thyroid gland, even the skeptics were convinced of the success of organ therapy.

From today's perspective, the effect can of course be explained by the hormone content of the preparations given. And back then, research also continued with hormone-rich tissues. In the Paris homeopathy laboratories, for example, various preparations were made from hormone glands, including placenta and mammary gland tissue.

Placenta was not only used in France, but also in Eastern European and Asian regions. A publication from the women's clinic in Saratov (Russia) on *Placenta as a Remedy in Folk Medicine* dates back to 1927. It describes the effect of placenta preparations used at the time: These remedies helped with weakness in labor, incomplete miscarriage and insufficient function of the mammary glands. According to this publication, placenta preparations were used with great success as a "galactogogum", a breast milk stimulant. The placenta was also used to treat postpartum illnesses. When exactly human placentas were used and when animal placentas were used is not always reported. However, wet nurses, for example, used extracts from sheep placentas to stimulate the production of breast milk. In parts of Kyrgyzstan, mothers were given an alcoholic extract of dried camel placenta to treat uterine bleeding after childbirth. It was therefore understandable for people at the time that animals instinctively ate their placenta after giving birth, as folk medicine was aware of its milk-promoting effect and also its effect on the uterus, stopping bleeding.

The trend towards the use of organ-containing preparations then continued into the post-war period. Dr. Möslein's doctorate is one of the testimonies to this.

The doctorate of Dr. Möslein

In 1949, Peter Möslein submitted his doctorate to the University of Jena with the title *Treatment of Secondary Amenorrhea with Fresh Embrocation from Glands (ovary and placenta)*. This doctoral thesis paints a picture of gynecology during and after the Second World War. As a result of bombing, the pharmaceutical industry was no longer able to produce medicines (and hormone preparations). People therefore looked for alternatives to treat amenorrhea - the cessation of menstruation. The physician Möslein describes how the number of patients with amenorrhea increased again in the final years of the Second World War. He refers to this as "wartime amenorrhea", as those affected did not have a disease of the reproductive organs, rather, the causes lay in malnutrition and war trauma. As a significant factor, he mentions mental stress; especially due to the hardships of refugee treks, the loss of home and livelihood, the separation and death of relatives and the great difficulties for refugees in their new home. The term "psychological amenorrhea" emerged, which was caused by difficulties of the post-war period, the uncertainty about death or life of the husband, the loss of livelihood and major changes in lifestyle. As the pharmaceutical industry was not in a position at this time to "even remotely provide the necessary preparations for a promising hormone therapy", another effective remedy had to be used: the fresh placenta. Möslein assumed that sex hormones were absorbed through the skin during external embrocation and rubbing.

> "The mature, expelled placenta was freed from the umbilical cord and amnion, minced in a meat grinder, mixed with a swelling mass, usually adulsion, and a small amount of an odor-correcting oil, e.g. rosemary oil. This preparation was [...] rubbed onto the broad surface of the back and the abdominal skin by means of a tapping massage."

The fact that the women's urine smelled of the rosemary oil used was cited as proof that the fat-soluble substances and hormones were absorbed through the skin.

Out of 78 women who were treated with this miraculous "cure", 64 women experienced success: Vaginal bleeding occurred during or afterwards the treatment. In 39 women, this bleeding was regular, i.e. the treatment led to the resumption of menstruation. It is interesting to note that among these 39 women there were also 6 patients who had not responded to previous hormone therapy with synthetic hormones.

Dr. Möslein saw the fresh gland treatment as a stimulus to the activity of the ovaries, which caused the endometrium to react. This would reinstate the rhythm of the female cycle again. The induced bleeding was a sure treatment success and had a very impressive effect on the women. It was also noted that those nurses who carried out the embrocation for a longer period of time experienced an increase in menses themselves.

> "The body thus receives [...] a mixture of hormones and vitamins in a natural state through the embrocation with fresh placenta. This enables the organism to use those of the supplied substances that are necessary to maintain or restore normal function."

And, to get ahead of ourselves: The use of placenta preparations for infertility is also described in Chinese medicine. Dr. Möslein was therefore able to confirm what had already been practiced in China centuries before: placenta as a "fertility remedy".

"Many world stars swear by it: Hormocenta!"

The German-Austrian actress Marika Rökk once used this slogan on television to advertise facial creme containing placenta. The commercial can still be found on YouTube today. But did all the international stars know what they were putting on their noses? Many older midwives still remember: "Sure, we used to collect the placentas after hospital births for the cosmetics industry. They were collected regularly and then they always gave us a few pennies for the coffee fund."

In the 1970s, the human placenta experienced a renaissance in its use in beauty products. Placenta extracts were also used in "Hormocenta" - and the benefits of the estrogens it contained for the skin were touted.

With the emergence of HIV, the commercial processing of placenta was stopped due to hygiene and infection regulations. Today, such products are therefore only available from sheep or with colostrum (the first milk) from cows. The alternative to hormone-containing cosmetics: becoming a midwife. We are sure that regularly sniffing placenta does something to the skin, as some of the ingredients are "volatile", i.e. they fly through the air and could be absorbed through the mucous membranes if inhaled. Most of the midwives we know therefore probably look fresh and rosy despite working regular night shifts - without any help from the cosmetics industry.

PLACENTA AS A REMEDY

If we want to understand placenta as a remedy from perspectives of integrative medicine, we need to take a brief look at these medical concepts. What does "integrative" actually mean? And does it need to be separated from modern medicine?

The medical perspective: dimensions of healing

by Sophia Johnson

Today's research-oriented pharmaceutical medicine is often reduced to the creation of facts: A special design is used to answer this or that question in a study. This often involves values, scores and measurable effects that can be expressed in figures. This two-dimensional thinking - key/lock, hormone/receptor - then also leaves its mark on the minds of medical professionals.

As a doctor, it once happened to me that I came to my oncology ward in the morning and sat down in front of the computer with a cup of coffee. I scrolled through the patient's lab results (thankfully, the students in their final year had already taken blood, so I didn't even have to enter the sick room to do this). There was a patient in room 301 who was seriously ill. In addition to acute leukemia, he had undergone major abdominal surgery. Then I saw his laboratory values: the leukocytes had not risen any further, the inflammation values were stable and even the kidney function had improved. Motivated, I took the medical records and started the ward round. But as I was about to enter his room, the nurse came out to tell me that the patient had just died. I hadn't expected that at all! What had happened in the time between the blood sample being taken and the ward round? Why didn't the blood analysis show the actual state of the patient's life?

For me, this experience was transformatory, as it made me realize that measured values do not express what *life* is. Of course, you might have to look for other laboratory parameters that are better suited to this question. But I don't know of any blood value that expresses a person's vital energy state. And as long as we doctors are on a two-dimensional search for factual truth, we are missing our perception of what is essential.

Seen from the perspective of Chinese medicine, this patient was already at the end of life, in absolute deficiency, the kidney energy was completely exhausted. But this has nothing to do with the kidney values of our laboratory medicine. In my view, integrative medicine concepts are more comprehensive because they share a philosophical understanding of life energy. And this energy refers not only to the metabolic level, but of course also to the soul. The body is not separated from the spirit. According to this integrative medical concept, the human being is also animated spiritually through inspiration (breathing).

In Chinese, there is a term for life energy: Qi. The aim of Chinese medicine treatment is to strengthen and harmonize this life energy. If Qi is blocked and cannot flow freely, this leads to symptoms of illness. And there is also a name for the mind in Chinese medicine: Shen. Shen corresponds to the human soul; it resides in the heart. Thus, not only the concept of vital energy, but also the concept of "spirit/soul" can be found in Chinese medicine.

Anthroposophical medicine also recognizes both the life energy (the so-called etheric body) and the soul (the so-called astral body) as essential parts of the human being. Illness occurs when these aspects of the human being are out of balance. This parallel can also be found in homeopathy: the aim of homeopathic treatment is to harmonize the life energy (known as dynamis). In addition to the specific physical symptoms, the mental and emotional symptoms are also considered to be important.

What all of these integrative concepts have in common is that they share an idea of "life energy", even if the terminology used is different. The therapeutic goal is to restore the harmonization and flow of life energy, not only on a physical level, but also in the soul and spirit. This keeps people healthy!

We therapists should therefore train ourselves in the perception of life energy, as this may enable us to learn more about the current state of our patients than a blood analysis can tell us. Will we ever find a laboratory parameter that can express the state of our vital energy and the clarity of our thoughts? Based on these considerations, it would be desirable to integrate this multidimensional thinking into modern medicine.

The integrative use of the placenta

As physicians, we are interested in the exact application of placenta as a remedy in the context of a particular integrative medical system. Because only then can we move from the realm of traditional experience to an exact concept of treatment, including symptoms, indication and therapy, according to each school of medical thought. This provides clarity for placenta therapy according to Chinese medicine, anthroposophical medicine or homeopathy. Although all these concepts have things in common – for example, the understanding of life energy (whether in the form of Qi, dynamis or ether-body) as the basis for the use of placenta as a remedy, the preparations and indications are quite different.

Chinese medicine

Chinese medicine is based on a philosophical view of the world and mankind, which is characterized by the constant change of the polarities yin and yang. What is referred to as life energy in the Western world is described in Chinese medicine as the aforementioned "Qi": a universal, flowing life force that constantly produces movement and change. According to Chinese understanding, Qi nourishes the blood and the organs. In the theory of disease, Qi can be, for example, deficient or stagnant, and thus produce various symptoms of illness. An anamnesis and diagnosis according to Chinese medicine is the basis for the individual prescription of remedies.

The use of powder from dried and/or steamed human placenta is described in Chinese pharmacopoeias. In the encyclopedia *Ben cao gang mu* by the 16th century physician Li Shizhen, dried, powdered placenta is combined with other medicinal plants. The use of this medicinal mixture is recommended for the following conditions: deficiency of Qi and blood combined with emaciation, exhaustion in women or insufficient milk production after childbirth as a result of Qi and blood exhaustion. Depending on the birth situation, women can show exactly these symptoms in the postpartum period. Placenta is described in this pharmacopoeia as an effective remedy for a whole range of ailments, especially for those specific to women. "It is outstanding, and cannot be compared to such categories as are metals, minerals, herbs and trees. Even the stupid will achieve effects when they use it."

In Chinese belief, at conception, the union of man and woman, the Qi of both mother and father is given to the developing child – as well as a portion of heavenly Qi. What distinguishes the placenta from all other medicinal drugs in Chinese medicine is that it is the carrier of prenatal Qi in the form of energy from the universe. From the philosophical consideration of the energetic power source placenta, one can understand the further applications of placenta. For men and women alike, the indications include: extreme exhaustion, deficiency states and epilepsy with fainting and loss of consciousness. Placenta is said to "pacify the heart and nourish the blood, it boosts the Qi and supplements the "essence".

The description "pills to supplement the kidney" must be understood from a broader understanding of kidney energy in Chinese medicine. This description does not only refer to the kidney and urinary tract, but also to the kidneys as carriers of "true Qi", the original energy. Placenta is therefore used as an effective, energizing remedy in the Chinese diagnosis of kidney weakness. The strengthening of kidney energy is the basis of the treatment of infertility and impotence, for which human placenta is indicated in women and men.

We know from a source from the 16th century that the ritual burial of the placenta was also very important in China. A respectful, traditional burial ensured the well-being of the newborn. It can therefore be assumed that traditional placenta preparations from pharmacies were only used for specific medical indications, but that mothers did not generally ingest their own placenta.

Even today, placenta is not only used as a remedy in Asia, but intensive research is also being carried out into therapy with placenta preparations. There is an entire area of scientific research in India and Japan dedicated to this. The positive effects of liquid extracts from human placenta on wound healing have been shown in studies, for example for wounds after operations, burns, chronic wounds or inflammation of the skin. The effect of dietary supplements made from pig placenta on sleep quality or menopausal complaints has also been assessed in clinical studies. Ancient knowledge, documented and handed down in Chinese pharmacopoeias, is thus becoming the subject of modern clinical research.

Homeopathy

The teaching of classical homeopathy goes back to the German doctor Samuel Hahnemann (1755–1843). In 18th century medicine, "therapy" was characterized by emetic and laxative cures, bloodletting and the prescription of sometimes highly toxic medicinal mixtures – but above all by superstition and ignorance. Out of necessity, in order to avoid having to use these sometimes dangerous, violent and risky therapies on his patients, Hahnemann developed a then modern, low-side-effect therapy of standardized dilution and potentization of medicinal drugs: homeopathy.

The understanding of health as an expression of life energy, which was widespread in Romantic medicine, is referred to as "dynamis" in homeopathy. The recognition of specific symptoms, the appropriate choice of the most suitable remedy and its repeated administration will lead to a gentle, rapid and lasting restoration of health. A series of standardized steps are necessary to turn an original substance into a homeopathic remedy. These processes are called "dynamization" or "potentization" which causes the revelation of the specific medicinal powers hidden in the original substance. Due to the potentization of homeopathic remedies, an area of action is addressed which, according to Hahnemann, not only has a direct influence on the life energy, but also on the mind.

As a pharmacist, Hahnemann had access to many different medicinal drugs. He tested them to find out what effects the respective remedy had on the healthy organism. Of course, the sometimes highly potent substances had to be used in appropriate, reduced doses and tested beforehand for purity and authenticity (for example, freshly squeezed plant juice). A healthy person who engaged in a moderate lifestyle and avoided any other drugs or remedies during the trial period took the medicinal substance over a specific period - and all symptoms that occurred in the meantime were documented in detail. This is how homeopathic reference books (*Materia Medica*) were created, in which the symptoms that occurred after taking medicinal drugs were collected.

Placenta humana is not listed in the *Materia Medica* of classical homeopathy. However, the symptoms of the proving of human placenta, which were collected by Kathy Biggs and Linda Gwillim in 2000, are included in today's pharmacopoeias. The starting substance was the placenta of a healthy woman without pregnancy complications after an uncomplicated spontaneous delivery. The pregnancy was without medication and there was no history of cancer or infection in the woman's family history. A liquid potentization was prepared from a small piece of this placenta. Healthy test subjects took the homeopathic remedy over a defined test period without knowing which medicine it was and recorded the symptoms they noticed.

Here is a selection of the symptoms that occurred in healthy people when taking potentized placenta: Anxiety, fear, apathy and emotionlessness, difficulty concentrating, a feeling of indifference, sadness, tearfulness, crying, swollen and firm breasts, a feeling of milk coming in. According to the Simili principle, namely to heal like with like, the symptoms listed above could lead to the prescription of homeopathic placenta remedies.

The increased sensory perception of the test participants was also noticeable during the homeopathic placenta intake: Vision was more intense and sharper and colors were perceived more vividly. A clear sensitivity to sounds was also described.

From a homeopathic point of view, placenta remedies belong to the "mother remedies". This group of remedies is indicated if the pregnancy or birth is the trigger for existing problems or symptoms. The "mother remedies" include Chorda umbilicalis (the umbilical cord), Amni liquor (the amniotic fluid), Placenta humana (already very well known to us), Vernix caseosa (the "cheese smear" or, to put it more nicely: baby's first skin protection cream), Oxytocinum (the important birth hormone) and Lac humanum (human breast milk).

Homeopathic medicine from placenta is prepared in accordance with the *European Pharmacopoeia*. The defined instructions of the *Homeopathic Pharmacopoeia* (HAB) are contained in this regulation, as applicable in Europe. Preparations made from placenta according to these instructions are called sarcodes, as the starting material is human tissue. Nosodes are preparations made from disease products. Therefore, the commonly used term placenta nosodes is misleading, as the placenta does not contain pathological material per se.

There are two variants of placenta remedies:

1. Placenta humana (not individualized): Remedies produced by manufacturers of homeopathic medicinal products
2. Individual placenta remedies: These are produced from the individual placenta in specialized pharmacies for the mother from her own placenta.

The latter is a current trend in Germany. The individually prepared placenta remedies are then used by mothers, sometimes for very broad indications for themselves or their child. The most common reason for the mother to take a homeopathic placenta remedy is a lactation disorder. It has also been documented that children are given placenta remedies by their mothers for colds, flatulence, problems falling asleep and neurodermatitis. The mothers observed an improvement in the symptoms, sometimes on the same day. From a homeopathic point of view, this does not seem entirely understandable, as there are certainly more suitable remedies for the respective clinical picture, depending on the main complaints and symptoms. After all, using placenta remedies like a watering can for a wide variety of complaints without a specific indication can of course lead to disappointment if there is no successful cure, but it can also be dangerous (for example for the child). A medical examination by an (homeopathic) health professional is therefore essential, especially in the case of persistent complaints. A detailed medical history and examination may lead to a more suitable choice of homeopathic medicine prescription.

Anthroposophical medicine

Anthroposophical medicine is based on a view of the human being that unites the material or physical body with an etheric body (vital body, growth and healing), and astral body (soul body, spiritual dynamics) and the ego or the "I" (the organization that guides the other bodies and shapes the individual human being, the actual spiritual center of each person).

From an anthroposophical point of view, the birth of the placenta is more than just the death of the mostly fetal tissue of the afterbirth. According to Rudolf Steiner, the founder of Anthroposophy, the organs surrounding the embryo (envelope organs) are formed by the "pre-earthly" human being. The placenta is the organ that relates to the warmth and to the "I" of the unborn child.

The Anthroposophist and evolutionary biologist Wolfgang Schad describes the placental birth as the formation of a partial corpse and the afterbirth as the "lost half of the human being". This loss accompanies people throughout their lives and creates the need for supplementation during the course of one's life through relationships with fellow human beings, the community, nature or faith. In his opinion, the afterbirth should be accorded the full dignity of human substance and thus, it should not be used for the production of remedies but rather be accorded a dignified burial. Schad describes the ingestion of one's own placenta after birth as "de facto cannibalism".

Christoph Zerm, long-time director of anthroposophical maternity clinic at the "Gemeinschaftskrankenhaus Herdecke", has studied the placenta intensively for many years. For him, the placenta is a kind of archetype of pedagogy. In the beginning, the placenta takes over all the tasks for the developing organism. The more the developing organism is able to take over functions itself during pregnancy, the more the placenta gradually withdraws. At birth, the placenta has fulfilled its task and dies.

Zerm sees the placenta as a representative of essential growth and formative forces that are involved in the development of the human organism during pregnancy. He therefore believes that it makes sense to also consider potentized preparations from the afterbirth in order to treat severe or chronic conditions in which there is a particular weakness of the growth and formative forces.

In anthroposophical medicine, remedies made from placenta are classified as organ preparations. These are also produced according to the regulations of the *Homeopathic Pharmacopoeia* and hardly differ from homeopathic medicines in terms of the manufacturing process. However, unlike in the two integrative medicine concepts described above, the placentas used for this purpose do not come from humans, but from cattle (Latin "bos") from biodynamic farms. A dignified inner attitude towards the animal is essential when retrieving a small piece of placenta tissue. Organ preparations of animal origin are intended to stimulate the etheric-body in particular. Liquid potentizations are produced from bovine placenta, they are given as an intradermal injection - or, for example in the case of children, can be drunk.

In anthroposophical medicine, the placenta is seen as a nourishing organ, both for the etheric-body and in relation to the soul and spirit. It strengthens the "I", which is associated with issues such as autonomy, self-regulation and inner independence. The warm quality of the potentized organ preparation and the information it contains about placental nutritional, excretory and educational functions can thus influence the whole organism as a restorative remedy.

The placenta in the individual integrative medical traditions

The use of the placenta as a remedy has a very long tradition in medicine. Although the various integrative therapy concepts are based on different philosophical views and concepts of man, there are interesting overlaps in the indication of placenta preparations, particularly the use in the postpartum period for lactation disorders and the general vitalization and strengthening of the organism. Depending on production and processing, however, the mode of action can also be directed at other levels of the human body: The higher the potency of the remedy, the more likely it is to address mental and spiritual aspects, such as mood symptoms. Here, a special sensitivity in the perception of the therapist and patient can help to observe healing tendencies beyond the purely physical.

Chinese medicine also describes placenta as sharpening vision and hearing. The same has been described in drug testing with homeopathic placenta remedies: Vision becomes more intense, sight sharper, hearing more sensitive. Anthroposophical medicine also uses placenta preparations for visual disorders and hearing loss.

Thus, taking placenta preparations reveals a phenomenon that pregnant women also describe: an increased sensitivity to external stimuli. This is quite cleverly conceived by nature, as it allows the expectant mother to perceive her environment with regard to the needs of the soon-to-arrive newborn. It is exciting that the placenta - even when it is still in the body - conveys this "feeling of being aware", a feeling of heightened consciousness.

Overview of the different medical concepts with the respective indication and processing of placenta preparations. All information relates to human placenta. The exception is Anthroposophic medicine: in this case organ preparations are of bovine origin.

Medical concept	**Indication**	**Preparation**
Chinese medicine	Deficiency of kidney qi, Deficiency of qi and blood, (lactation disorders, exhaustion, infertility)	Placenta humana, Steamed and/or dehydrated placental tissue combined with medicinal plants
Homeopathy	Lactation disorders, mental symptoms (anxiety, sadness), disturbance of the mother-child bonding	Placenta humana (individual remedy), mother tincture and potentizations (e.g. D-potencies, C-potencies)
Anthroposophic medicine	Therapeutic influence on the ego-organization (ego disorder), stimulate the etheric body	Placenta bovis, Potencies D5-D30, Liquid dilution for injection or drinking
Use in obstetrics	**Indication**	**Preparation**
Traditional midwifery	To give during "difficult births", to expel the afterbirth	Placenta humana, raw dried placental tissue
Human maternal placentophagy	Postpartum depression, lactation disorders, Fatigue, acceleration of recovery from birth	Placenta humana (individual production), Placenta pieces, raw; steamed or raw dried tissue, packed in capsules

PLACENTOPHAGY

A clarification of terms

The vernacular has coined an exciting term for the placenta: "the mother's cake". Our own children, who had never seen a placenta at that time, imagined it to be something very tasty. Probably a mixture of tart and chocolate cake. The reality of seeing a placenta for the first time was disappointing for them.

Placenta comes from the Latin "placenta" and means flat cake. Perhaps it is also related to the Latin verb "placere", which means to please or to satisfy? If so, the idea of tasting is not particularly far-fetched. However, if you search for a word that describes placenta tasting, you will come across the term "placentophagy".

Placentophagy is a scientific term that is used worldwide. The derivation of the word is relatively simple: we already know placenta. "Phag" is a suffix that comes from Greek and is derived from the word "phagein" - "to devour, to eat". Placentophagy could therefore be translated as placenta consumption.

Sometimes remedies are made from a placenta that are not only taken by the mother. In some cultures, the newborn's family, for example a sick sibling, also receives some of the "placenta". This is known as human placentophagy. However, if the mother ingests her own, very individual placenta, this is described scientifically as "human maternal placentophagy", i.e. the consumption of the placenta by the mother.

So, having sorted out the terms, now we can go into detail.

Placentophagy in the animal kingdom

What we know: Almost all of them do it. At least mammals do. With very few exceptions, such as camels and whales. The latter because they prefer to devote themselves to their offspring rather than swim after their placenta – sounds very sensible!

Placentophagy can be observed among herbivores and carnivores, nest feeders and nest hoppers. So even cows that actually only feed on plants will eat their placenta if they are allowed to. Two hypotheses attempt to explain this behavior: the assumption of nest cleanliness and that of enemy avoidance. However, these hypotheses are contestable. For example, suckling animals that give birth in trees (such as tree squirrels or monkeys) consume their placenta instead of throwing it out of the nest for reasons of cleanliness. They even climb down from the tree to retrieve the placenta if it has fallen during birth. And whether "enemy avoidance" is really the reason for placentophagy? Seems doubtful, as even predators such as lionesses, which are at the top of the food chain and have no other predators to fear, eat their placenta.

Or is it simply hunger? In an experiment, rodents were given a choice between liver, beef, pork and placenta after birth – what did they chose? The placenta! Anthropologist Daniel Benyshek therefore suspects that there must be something very special, something specific that makes the animals consume the placenta. But what this is, we can only hypothesize so far.

Nature is not wasteful

by Sophia Johnson

I once attended a rather dramatic rabbit birth in which the baby rabbits did not survive. Fortunately, the mother rabbit did not die during the birth – when I checked on her a short time later, she had eaten both the afterbirth and the stillbirths. When I later told this story to an older doctor friend of mine, he simply said: "Nature is not wasteful."

Effects in the animal kingdom

There are many studies from the animal kingdom that show the effects of placentophagy. We are particularly fascinated by the collared peccaries (Tayassu tajaku). These are small wild pigs that are mainly native to North and South America. A zoologist in Zurich observed the following in a group of animals in captivity: After giving birth, the peccary mother recovered. Breastfeeding was not done by her, but by wet nurses: not yet fully grown, so-called subadult females from the group. These are usually only a few months old themselves and sometimes still suckle from their own foster mothers. In addition, these young wet nurses have not experienced pregnancy themselves. But they engaged in placentophagy after birth. Apparently, eating the foreign placenta, together with the stimulation of the teats by the newborns when sucking, triggers milk production in these animals. This ensures breastfeeding of the peccary offspring independently of their own mother. Some further findings have been made in rodents. For example, the ingestion of placenta leads to altered prolactin and progesterone levels in the blood of rats. Further studies show that neurochemical factors in the placenta increase attraction to the newborn and affection (i.e. maternal behavior).

Pain-free through placentophagy!?

A research team led by Mark Kristal was also able to make another exciting observation: placentophagy reduces anxious behavior in mice and apparently has an analgesic effect. In practical terms, this means that mice that have eaten their placenta can be pinched in the tail for longer than mice that have not eaten their placenta.

A placenta-specific "factor" is currently captivating the attention of scientists: POEF – the "placental opioid enhancing factor". The term "factor" is a bit of a misnomer, as it is not known exactly what this factor actually is: It is too large to be a hormone. POEF is therefore initially characterized as a heat-stable molecule – in other words, as a small chemical particle.

To understand the significance of POEF, you need a little background knowledge: There are a lot of nerve cells in the human brain that produce neurotransmitters (for example endorphins). The entirety of nerve cells and the messenger substances they produce, which run through our brain structures, is called the endogenous opioid system. Or, translated: the body's own pain and stress processing system. The entirety of the messenger substances is called endogenous opioids or endogenous pain-relieving substances. In addition to endorphins, they also include enkephalins and dynorphins.

Endogenous opioids are the body's natural response to pain, stress and anxiety. They are also released at birth and produced by the placenta during pregnancy. POEF is also part of the endogenous opioid system as a factor that induces pain relief after placental consumption as described above in the mouse model.

When the body's own pain system is stimulated by opioids, POEF ensures that the opioid effect is intensified and even more pain receptors are activated. This molecule could therefore be described as a booster of the body's own pain relief. We are very excited to see what research in this area will uncover in the coming years: Do human placentas also have a POEF molecule?

Maternal placenta ingestion

We now know that mammals eat their placenta. And it is very likely that our ancestors, the prehistoric humans, also ate their placenta, but we will come back to this later. Quite a few postpartum women today are once again consuming their placenta. We know this from midwives who care for women in the postpartum period. However, we cannot yet say how common human maternal placentophagy is in Germany. It is not always talked about openly and this topic is sometimes socially taboo or judged in a derogatory way. But regardless of this, women do placentophagy without talking much about it. It would be interesting to collect and analyze data on placentophagy as part of the midwife's postpartum visit. This was done in America: The data from 23,242 out-of-hospital births was scientifically analyzed. This showed that almost a third of all women who gave birth in birth centers or at home in the USA had their placenta processed into capsules and then ingested them. There is even a term for this: placenta encapsulation. These capsules are supposed to be *the* miracle pills for the postpartum period!

"Placenta capsules": the miracle pills for the postpartum period?

It's actually a really simple and therefore ingenious idea: in order to get the processed placental tissue back into the mother, it has to be adapted to our current practices: Dried placental tissue is pulverized and filled into empty capsules (these are available in gelatin or also plant-based form, even fruit-flavored). These capsules can then be conveniently consumed as a dietary supplement, similar to a vitamin, lactobacillus or magnesium capsule.

There is now a steadily increasing number of placenta service organizations in the United States. In 2006 Jodie Selander was the first woman to set up a placenta encapsulation business there with PBi (Placenta Benefits). Since then, she has been training placenta encapsulation specialists. Placenta encapsulation is not only widespread in the US, but also in the UK, Australia, Spain and parts of South America. In Germany, too, there are now similar offers, including placenta encapsulation from doulas.

When ordering, the customer can choose how the placenta is to be processed: either dried and then filled into capsules or first steamed, then dried and then filled into capsules. This "placenta encapsulation" service can be purchased if a woman does not want to process the placenta herself. The placenta is then collected after the birth by a certified encapsulation specialist and returned in capsule form after one or two days. Depending on the provider, you can also order a wide variety of products made from placenta: Placenta tincture, placenta essence, placenta tea, placenta ointment, placenta cream, placenta truffles, placenta smoothies or even the very individual placenta Bolognese ... And for all those who like to have their placenta hanging in the living room, there is also the "placenta print" to order – a work of art with the imprint of your own placenta. Very creative!

Modern maternal placentophagy

It is not entirely clear how this trend of women consuming their own placenta after giving birth came about. The American pathologist William Ober discussed placentophagy in one of his essays in 1968, not in a scientific sense, but as a partly amused observation of this exotic and primitive behavior.

A little earlier, around 1960, a movement formed in the USA against the mechanized and increasingly male-dominated field of obstetric medicine, which was characterized by interventions during birth process. At this time, women began to desire a self-determined, responsible birth. As a result, the number of midwife-assisted out-of-hospital births increased. At the same time, there was also a greater focus on natural birth.

The feminist movement had made great strides after the Second World War and issues such as political equality, the compatibility of motherhood and work (especially during the war, many women were irreplaceable as workers), sexual freedom and, of course, the invention of the "pill" gave the women's movement a real boost. A public discussion about homosexuality and the monogamous marriage construct began. The hippie movement emerged in the San Francisco area, partly as a provocation of staid norms. With mottos such as "Make love not war", the hippies made statements for peace, self-determination, creativity and sexual freedom.

The placentophagy hype may have started in the USA in the 1970s and originated in an article in *Rolling Stone* in 1972. In this world-famous music magazine, a young woman reported about her home birth, accompanied by a midwife and her partner, in the company of her friends, including children and a dog. Marijuana was smoked during the birth, and afterwards the placenta was steamed as a dish to be eaten. The article certainly caused a stir, set an example for free birth and was possibly the prelude to placenta as a remedy in the USA.

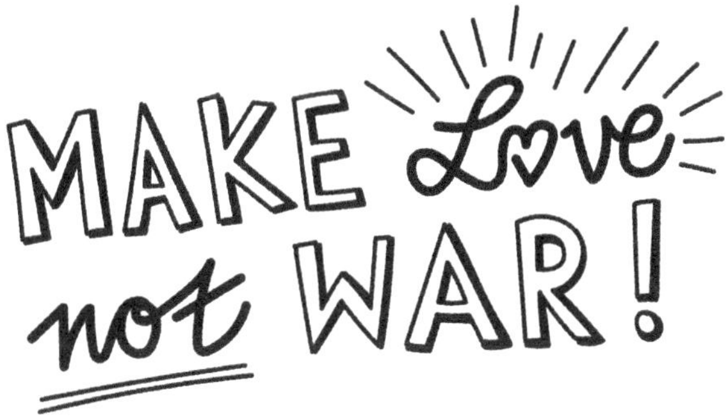

The placenta as a social media star

The placenta made it big in 2015 together with reality starlet Kim Kardashian. When the American made it public that she was taking her placenta in the form of capsules to prevent postpartum depression, the German tabloid press threw itself at the easy target. Fascination, disgust and condemnation characterized the reporting. It would have been nicer to use this media hype for focusing on the health of postpartum women: This would require headlines that identify the real problem, namely the fear of postpartum depression, instead of judging it negatively. After all, most women do not consume placenta for reasons of style, trend or beauty, but out of a desire to stabilize their emotional situation and not ride an emotional rollercoaster after having a newborn.

Of course, you also have to look at who wrote all these highly unhelpful articles: Man or woman, with or without children, with what cultural and political background, personal attitude etc. - and continue to come to terms with the fact that these written words are now out in the world, even if they are not particularly clever or sensitively articulated.

The placenta is presented in a much more balanced way on internet platforms. Especially in mothers' forums, where topics relating to pregnancy, birth and the first years of childhood are discussed, the placenta is a star. When women share their experiences with placenta as a remedy online, they are respectful of the individual experiences described. Positive reports of placentophagy predominate, with placenta most commonly taken as a capsule. Negative reports are often dominated by descriptions of disgust or discomfort during ingestion, but are rare compared to the positive experiences. It is clear that these women are not concerned with standardized medical guidelines on the subject of health in the postpartum period, but with their individual experience using their very own placenta as a remedy. The focus is on the mother's personal decision, her autonomy over her own body and freedom of action.

Placentophagy from an anthropological perspective

Why do women use their own placenta? Since 2010, anthropologists at the University of Las Vegas, Nevada (United States) have been investigating this question and researching the behavior of maternal placenta ingestion - above all Sharon Young and Daniel Benyshek.

In a cross-cultural study, they were able to prove that the placenta is used ritually in many ethnic groups and is generally known as a remedy. For maternal placenta ingestion, there was only one piece of evidence from 1986: a Mexican-American mother roasted her placenta after giving birth and felt incredibly full of energy after ingesting it.

In 2013, the anthropologists created a questionnaire for mothers who engaged in placentophagy. This study enabled the researchers to work out the motives and experiences: Most women took their placenta in the form of capsules. They wanted to stimulate milk production, stabilize their mood and avoid depression, as well as alleviate pain, support postnatal recovery and increase their energy levels in the postpartum period. This seems to work well. When asked about their experiences, 95% of the women said it was a good to very good experience and 98% of them would use placenta again.

The American data shows that women are predominantly "white", better educated than the average and wealthy. This example shows once again how much money and education influence health. We urgently need more equal opportunities so that not only white, educated women can make use of knowledge about the placenta as a remedy!

The fire hypothesis

What is also very interesting from an anthropological point of view is the question of whether placentophagy is a human behavior and whether this behavior pattern has changed in the course of biological evolution. How does Homo sapiens differ from its closest relatives - the primates?

Researcher Sharon Young assumes that prehistoric humans ate their placenta - as almost all mammals do. But what factors led Homo sapiens to stop that at some point? Was there a good reason for placentophagy to disappear from human behavior in the course of biological evolution?

"Purifying selection" is an term from evolutionary biology and means discarding harmful, inherited traits. (How nice it would sometimes be to simply stow away negative traits in a box like old clothes ...) In this case, however, it means that behavioral patterns that are unfavorable for a species should not be passed on to the next generation.

This is where Sharon Young's fire hypothesis comes into play: the controlled use of fire by humans began around 1.9 million to 250.000 years ago. The anthropologist assumes that women in particular guarded the fire and inhaled smoke over a long period of time. Theoretically, cadmium and particulate matter could have accumulated in the placenta, which - after ingestion - had a negative effect on fertility. However, from an archaeological point of view, we can only speculate as to whether pregnant women primarily guarded the fire or took on completely different tasks.

We now know from studies that the level of cadmium in the placenta is higher in smokers than in non-smokers. It is also known that in non-smokers, the potentially toxic elements can only be measured in very low doses (see chapter *Trace elements in placental tissue*). From today's perspective, one could therefore conclude that for a non-smoker who is not exposed to smoke from an open fire for many hours a day, cadmium poisoning through placentophagy is unlikely.

So perhaps the fire hypothesis remains just a hypothesis?

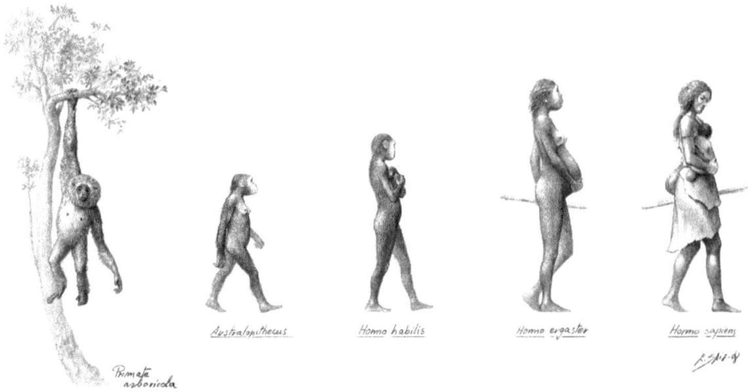

On the loss of human placentophagy ...

We can only speculate about the reasons why placentophagy is not (or no longer) practiced by us humans as a rule. But we are very interested in this question and have repeatedly discussed various theories. However, clear evidence is hard to find. We assume that there was not just one cause, such as the use of fire by humans, but that many human-historical factors and cultural developments played a role.

Perhaps there was a very practical aspect that superseded placentophagy. Women can be very exhausted, weak and above all hungry after giving birth. But what if there is no permanent access to food, no full fridge nearby, nothing to satisfy postpartum hunger? Is it then not understandable that the mother of the Stone Age roasted the "mother´s cake" over the fire after giving birth? Was this behavior abandoned when there was sufficient food available?

However, it is also possible that placentophagy was lost for other reasons and in many small steps over the course of thousands of years. There were probably great temporal and local differences in how, when and whether placentophagy was still or no longer practiced by various ethnic groups. Nature is dynamic, and so are societies.

Over the centuries, the rules of human life changed fundamentally as people settled down and made the transition from a nomadic "hunter-gatherer culture" to a more settled agricultural society. Biologist Meike Stoverock has put forward the fascinating theory that a key aspect of these changes was the loss of *female choice*. *Female choice* describes (in very simplified terms) a biological principle: the choice of sexual partner by the female, in humans of course by the woman. In Stoverock's opinion, the loss of *female choice* had enormous consequences for both sexes: "men" wanted to pass on their property to their actual biological descendants. With ownership, power and coercion emerged, and with them, defense mechanisms. In some cultures, monogamy became the norm and was now a "life sentence". And it was not only women who became unfree as a result, but also many men who were dominated by a few powerful male leaders. It is possible that in the course of these fundamental social changes, the behaviors of placentophagy were also completely or partially lost. The loss of *female choice* paved the way for many further steps in cultural evolution, which is interwoven with the development of different religions. We know from various sources that in Christianity, rituals involving the placenta were forbidden as "pagan" and corresponding customs were increasingly suppressed. Could it be that religions played a role in the disappearance of placentophagy much earlier?

There is one place in the Old Testament where placentophagy is mentioned, namely the prophetic warning from the fifth book of Moses, which contains exhortations to obey the word of God: "The finest woman among you, who has been carried around in a litter all her life, will eat her afterbirth and her newborn child in secret. She will not be willing to share with her husband or her other children because she would starve. So great will be the distress when your enemies besiege your cities." (Deuteronomy 28:57) We interpret this passage as a drastic warning of a famine that will come upon the people if God's commandments are not obeyed. The woman is portrayed as a selfish "child and placenta-eating female". Placentophagy is obviously already taboo in the Old Testament. But was it so well-known back then that placentophagy had to be mentioned in the Bible with a negative connotation?

We cannot make a blanket assumption that placentophagy has been lost across cultures, and we can only speculate that there may be native ethnic groups in which it has persisted. As we have already shown, knowledge of the placenta as a remedy was and still is widespread in Europe. However, we have found very few sources on maternal placentophagy. Perhaps this is because placentophagy was of little importance from a male perspective and so no written evidence of it is available because correspondence and documents were rarely written and left behind by women. It is also possible that these sources on maternal placenta ingestion do not actually exist. Or we just don't know about them because they are not understood by today's scientists. Because today – at least in our culture – hardly anyone knows about this behavior. Perhaps the tradition of circulating "female wisdom" within a social group was lost over generations. And maybe the persecution of so-called witches in the early modern period also played a role in the loss of knowledge about the placenta and its effects.

It is documented that outside Europe, colonization (combined with Christianization) had a clear influence on the demise of ritual acts surrounding the placenta. Was this perhaps a further influence on the consumption of the placenta?

With the beginning of territorial conquests and the discovery of new, previously unknown civilizations, placentophagy was occasionally mentioned by travelers. For example, there is a source from the Calvinist clergyman, traveler and writer Jean de Léry from 1556, in which he describes that the indigenous population in Brazil ate the afterbirth "like an animal" as soon as the mother expelled it. Placentophagy is seen as a primitive behavior of non-civilized cultures and therefore no longer seems to have been a common practice in Europe at this time.

However, there is also a letter from Leopold Mozart dated February 9, 1756, in which he wrote about the birth of his son Wolfgang Amadeus in Salzburg: "Incidentally, I would like to inform you that on January 27, at 8 o'clock in the evening, my wife was happily delivered of a boy, but the afterbirth had to be taken away. She was therefore surprisingly weak. But now, thank God, both child and mother are well." Could we conclude from this reference, that in 18th

century Austria, women were given their own placenta to strengthen themselves after giving birth? And even in highly educated circles? We know that Leopold Mozart, besides being a composer and musician, was well versed in medicine and had a broad knowledge of remedies, nutrition (during pregnancy), menstruation and postpartum problems. We can only speculate as to why Anna Maria Mozart's afterbirth was taken away. But perhaps the relative contraindications were already known at the time and maybe, for example, placentas from births with green amniotic fluid were not used, if the child was stressed during birth and had passed meconium into the amniotic fluid. In fact, you can still meet midwives from Austria today who remember: "Of course, we used to give women their placenta dried and ground as a tonic in the postpartum period."

In the 19th century, industrialization with its technical innovations such as the railroad and the engineering and mining industries also shaped our ideas in favor of a "mechanistic" view of the world. This functional approach was also adopted in medicine and the natural sciences. Modern science was introduced by men and was dominated by two-dimensional patterns of thought and explanation. This also had an impact on obstetrics. In the middle of the 20th century, births were transferred from the home environment to the clinic. The natural process became a standardized medical procedure. Midwives became subordinate to doctors. In many parts of France, when the placenta was still placed on the mother's breast after the birth, midwives were severely condemned by doctors for this ritual. Was the supposed progress of humanity a step backwards for the importance of the placenta?

But how can we explain the rediscovery of the placenta as a remedy in the Western world? Was the re-emergence of placentophagy at the same time as sexual liberation in the late 1960s perhaps also a rebellion against the demise of *female choice* and an attempt to break the social conventions of that time? And was this also an attempt by women to free themselves from the domestic and mental isolation that has characterized social coexistence for many millennia? Is the modern statement "My body, my choice" the answer to the loss of *female choice*?

To conclude with the question of whether the loss of placentophagy was a "purifying selection": Perhaps the exact opposite is the case. Perhaps we even need to ask whether "non-ingestion" of the placenta is a risk factor for the health status of postpartum women. After all, thinking scientifically means questioning the status quo and regularly changing our view of things as well as our perspective.

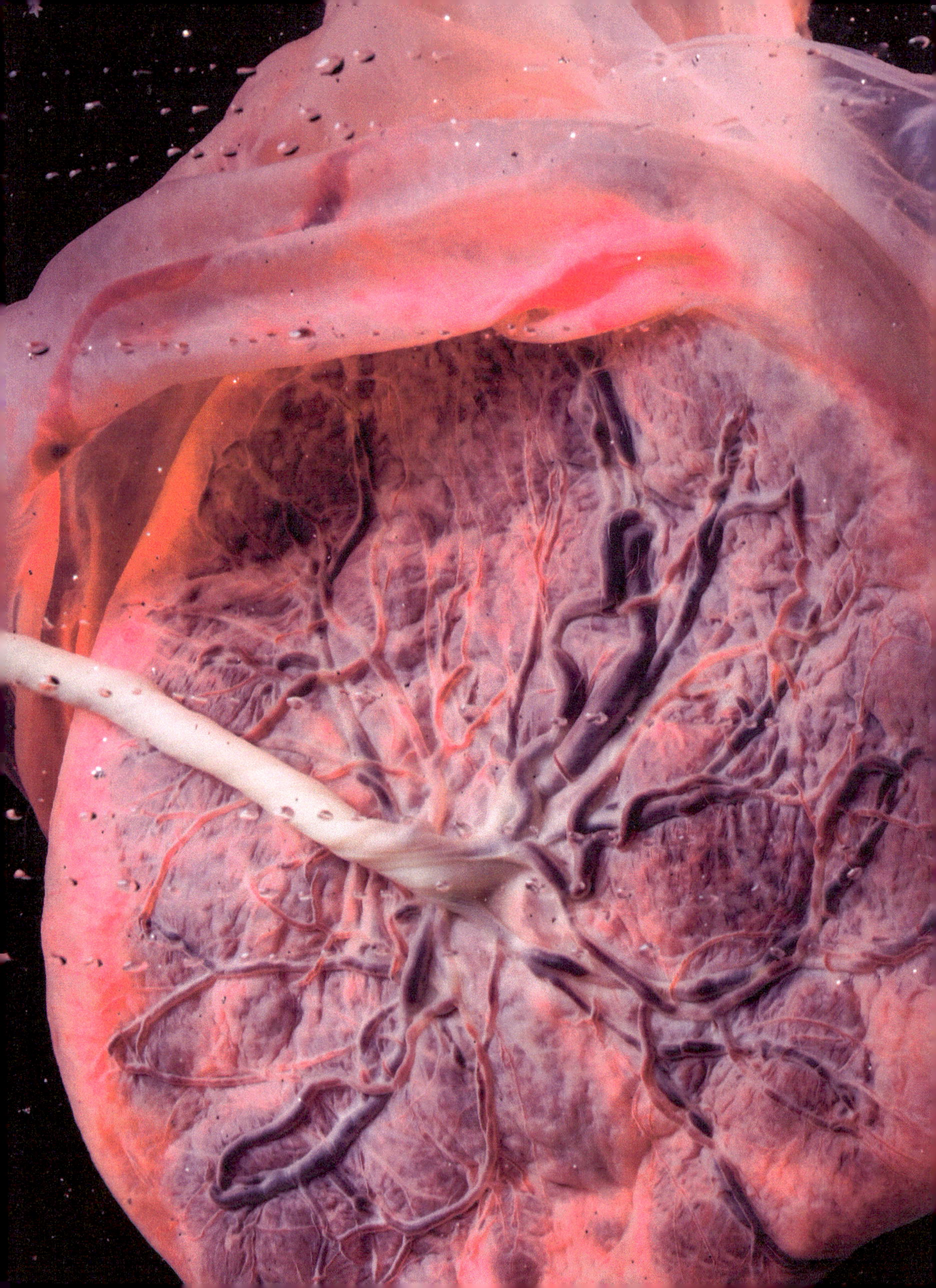

DRUG OR FOOD?

We have already outlined that the placenta was traditionally used as a remedy. At that time, it was included in pharmacopoeias without institutional approval. But is the placenta legally a medicine at all? Or just "a piece of meat" and therefore a foodstuff? This is of course an interesting question, especially when the placenta is processed into capsules. After all, this determines which rules the placenta products are subject to and what they can be compared with.

In Germany the Federal Institute for Risk Assessment regularly checks food for safety. The placenta as food? That would be human tissue, which is not eaten for ethical reasons ... But theoretically you could simply compare placenta with any other organ (of animal origin) on the butcher's counter: Tongue (optionally from cattle), liver (from the unfortunate pig - the detoxification organ certainly contains a colorful mix of pharmaceuticals), slaughtering blood (prepared into cooked sausage) ...

Pigs have had an average of six cycles of antibiotics by the time they are slaughtered - and what about placenta? In hardly any other stage of life do women nourish themselves as consciously as during pregnancy and avoid "poisons" and medication. But the comparison is admittedly skewed.

Nevertheless, it remains unclear how placenta can be categorized. If it is processed into lasagna (following various YouTube cooking recipes), it would probably be classified as food. But what about the capsules?

In comparison with the production of homeopathic placenta medicine by pharmacies, "placenta encapsulation" is based on traditional applications that describe the drying and pulverization of placental tissue. The dried tissue is filled into empty capsules. When it comes to the definition of these capsules made from placenta, things get quite complicated. Because then you have to distinguish what it is: A medicine? A food supplement? Human tissue or a tissue preparation?

Depending on the definition, very different regulations apply to placenta preparations in Germany. If you take a substance with a "healing promise", it falls under the German Medicinal Products Act (AMG). And as soon as any active ingredient is declared a medicinal product in Germany, the Federal Institute for Drugs and Medical Devices (Bfarm) is responsible as an institution of the federal government. This department defines that placenta capsules fall under "individual production" and that if you want to produce them for others, you need a manufacturing license from the respective state authority of the federal state. If women experiment with their own placenta in their kitchen and make the capsules for themselves, they obviously do not need permission to do so.

In the US, the debate about the definition of placenta has been going on for some time, as processing into capsules is much more widespread there than in Germany.

In a paper published by Greer Donley from Pittsburgh University School of law, there are some clever ideas on the future classification of the capsules produced during "placenta encapsulation". According to this source, they should be declared both as food supplements and as human tissue. The author states, that the use of placenta in the US should be regulated by the FDA (United States Food and Drug Administration) – but the FDA has not yet created any clear definitions.

In the UK, the equivalent to the FDA is the Food Standard Agency (FSA). In 2020, this authority declared the processing of placenta into capsules as a "food preparation business". Accordingly, the food safety rules apply to the service of manufacturing placenta capsules there.

On the one hand, this product monitoring is of course important to ensure safe use and protect consumers from potential risks. On the other hand, when it comes to sensitive issues such as pregnancy and childbirth, there is also a risk of over-regulation and the associated risk of interfering with a woman's right to self-determination. A barrier of regulations is then created and women's right to co-determination is disregarded. All regulations should therefore always focus on meaningful protection of female consumers and appropriate risk assessment.

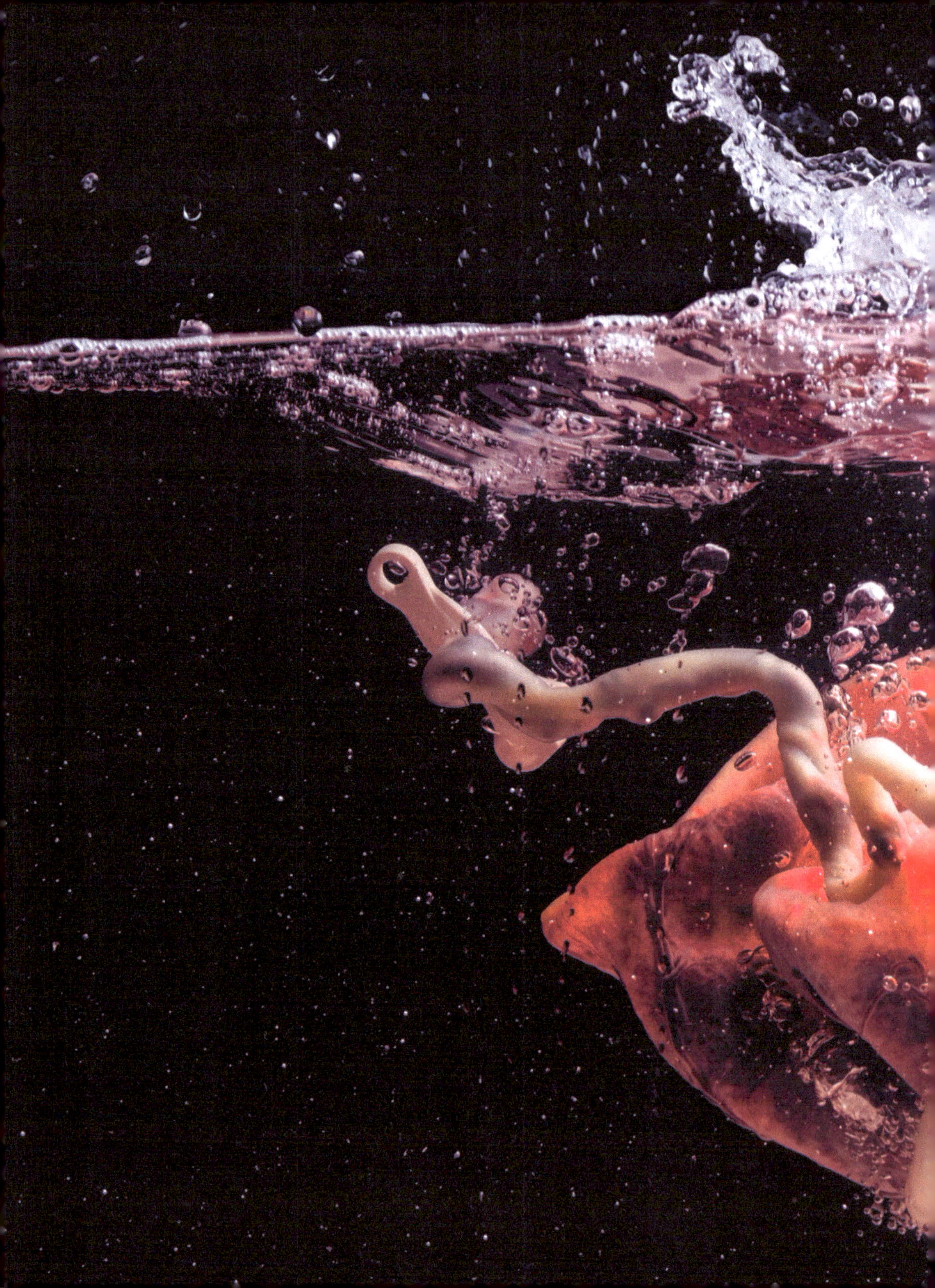

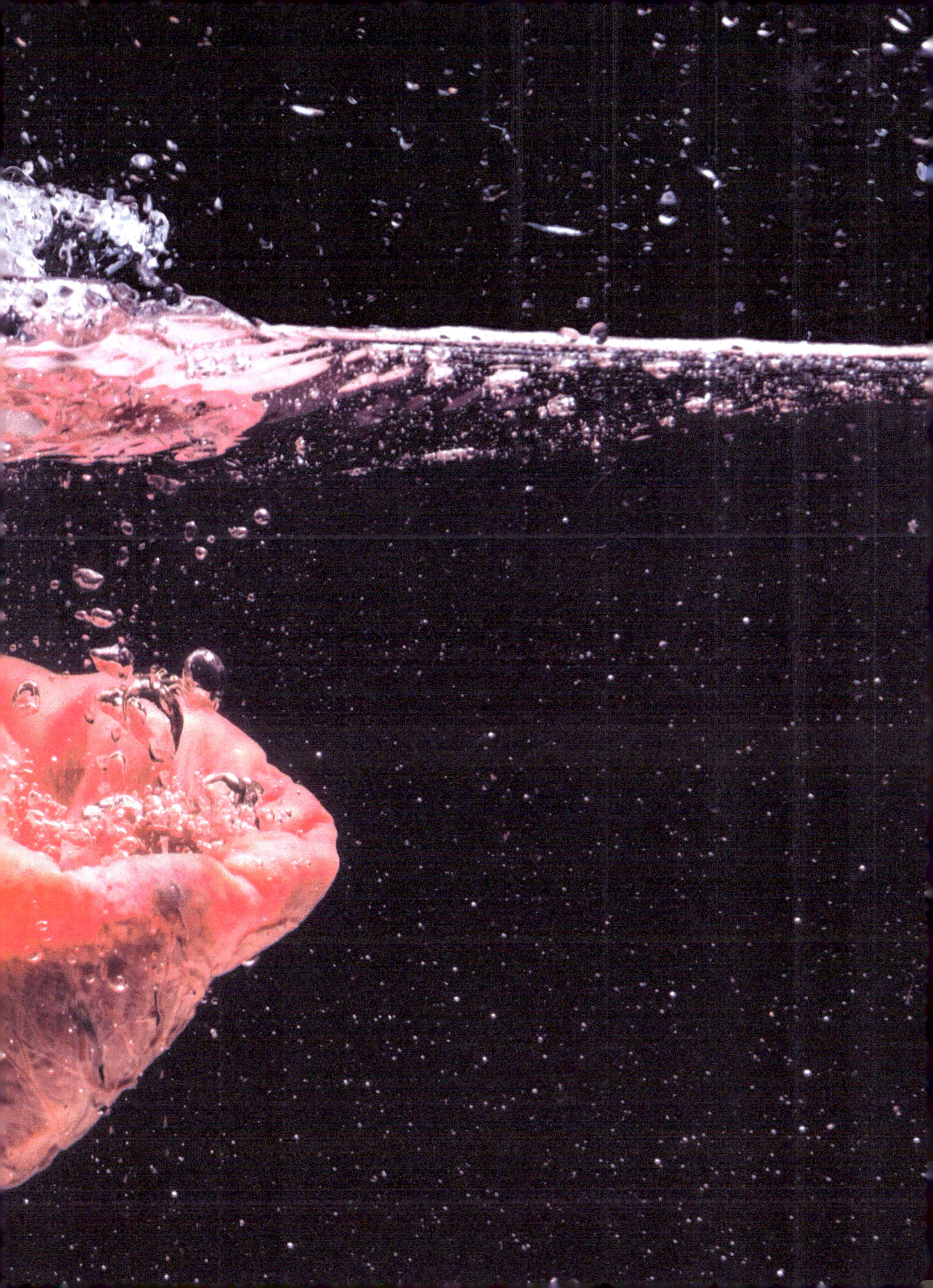

… OF COURSE, THE MOTHER CAN DECIDE!

If a woman is nowadays faced with the choice between placenta burial, placenta remedies or disposal in the trash, it should at least be clarified beforehand who actually owns the placenta and who is allowed to dispose of it. And since, genetically speaking, the majority of the placenta is infantile, shouldn't the newborn decide?

The placenta contains both maternal and fetal cells - and it is difficult to separate them out in order to define whose property it is … But even if the macroscopic separation of maternal and fetal tissue is not possible, from a purely legal point of view (referring to German law) it would be permissible: The maternal part of the placenta belongs to the mother and must therefore be handed over to her by the maternity clinic. According to these principles, the fetal part of the placenta belongs to the newborn (as does the umbilical cord), because it belongs to the newborn's body. However, as the newborn is not yet legally competent, it is not yet able to decide for itself what should happen to its share of the placenta. Therefore, the legal guardians (usually the parents) can decide in the interests of the child and, in this capacity, demand that the clinic hand over the entire placenta. One could also conclude that if the mother uses her own placenta to make a remedy for the puerperium and feels better as a result, the newborn naturally also benefits from this (she acts in the interest of the newborn).

Fortunately, the reality in German clinics is not quite as complicated as the legal classification of the issue: when you arrive in the delivery room, you tell the midwives that you would like to take the placenta with you after the birth. It is best to bring a clean, well-sealed container with you, then the placenta will usually be given to you. Of course, in exceptional situations it may be that the placenta needs to be examined further in the pathology department or that it ends up in the hospital waste disposal unit in the rush of an emergency caesarean section, contrary to the mother's wishes. But this very rarely happens.

The situation is different for example in the US, where the guidelines for handing over the placenta vary from state to state and only 61% of all clinics hand over to mothers their own placenta on request. There, too, the placenta is regarded as organ waste that could theoretically be infectious. However, the microorganisms on placental tissue are generally harmless, as we have been able to prove in our research, which we will come to in a moment. But of course, despite all the euphoria about placenta use, we must not forget that this is human tissue, which is by no means sterile. After birth, the placenta should therefore be cooled quickly so that it does not become a real "biohazard". This is because an unchilled organ, like a piece of raw meat, can easily spoil.

It is important to know that a placenta must be disposed of properly! In Germany this is regulated at municipal level by the local waste disposal authorities. In the case of home births or out-of-hospital births, the parents are informed accordingly by the midwife and must sign a document that states that they understand the rules of placenta disposal. They may then, for example, bury the placenta on their own property and plant a tree on it. It is not only for hygienic reasons that you must adhere to the guidelines when disposing of the placenta. There have already been cases of insufficiently buried umbilical cords being dug up by animals in municipal parks and the police being called in order to rule out a crime.

The question of disposal is of course superfluous if the placenta is to be used as a remedy and is therefore stored in the freezer or refrigerator. If the mother makes capsules from the placenta or has them made, there is usually nothing left of the tissue. To make homeopathic medicine from your own placenta, you only need a small piece, which is often cut out by the midwives in the delivery room. During births in hospital, the placenta is then disposed of as medical waste.

However, if there is no particular personal interest in your own placenta, you can also donate it for research purposes to a local university hospital with associated research laboratory.

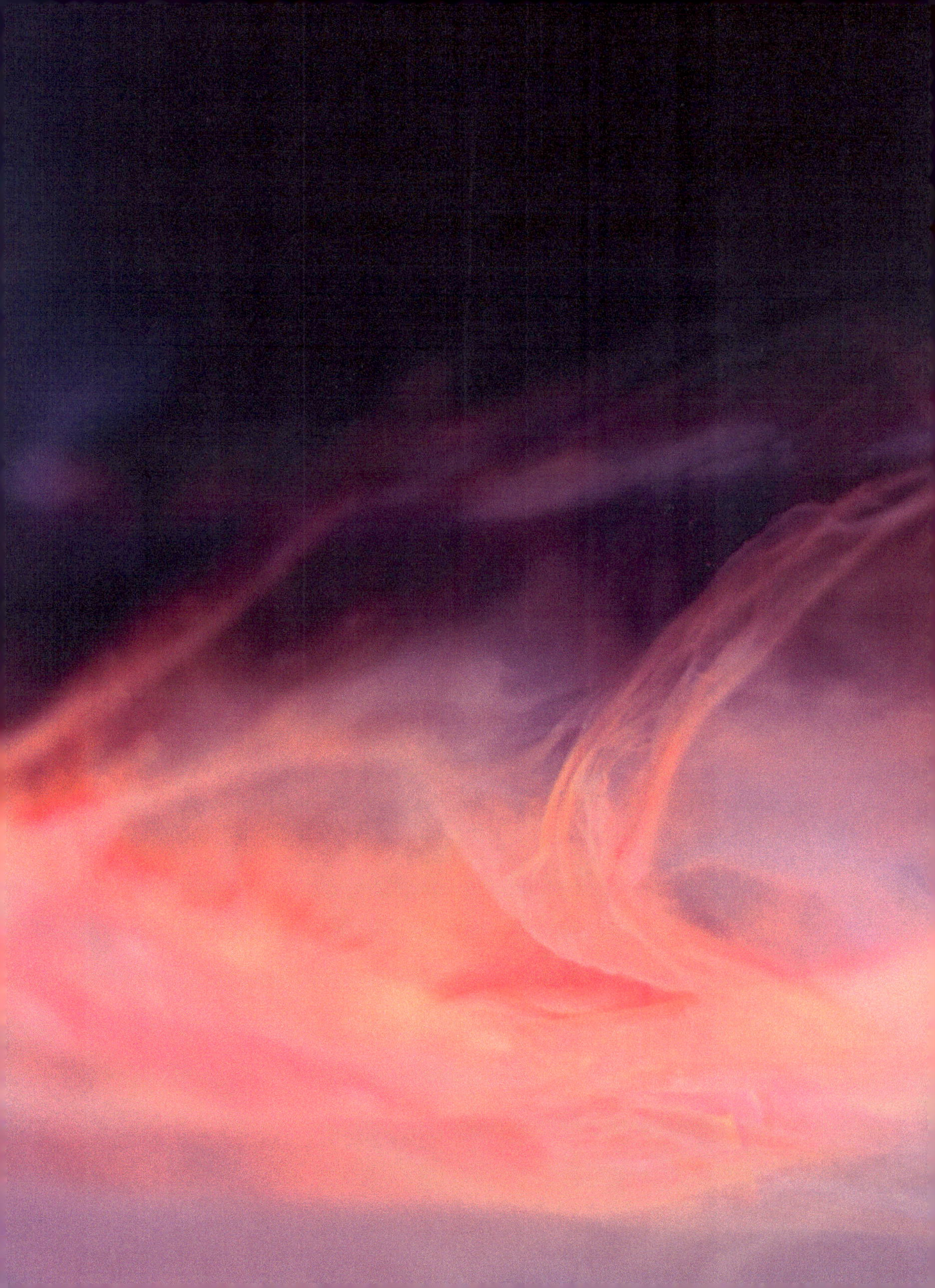

THE PLACENTA AS A RESEARCH OBJECT

The special thing about our research in the placenta lab is that we have the opportunity to experiment with a healthy, complete and fresh organ. For example, a few minutes after the placenta is born, we can create simulated maternal and fetal circulations in the laboratory and keep the placenta alive for a few more hours. This model of human placenta perfusion is only established in a few research groups in Europe and worldwide. This method is also known as ex-vivo perfusion (translated: taken from life and artificially supplied with fluid). The placenta perfusion research model is used to investigate whether a drug reaches the child via the placenta. We can use this model to test whether certain substances are transferred from the mother's side to the child's side. Indirectly, a transfer to the child's side also describes a contact on the part of the unborn child with the investigated substance. For many medicines or particles, it is not desirable for them to reach the unborn child. However, it has been shown in recent years that, for example, nanoparticles, microplastics and small carbon black particles can cross the placental barrier.

However, with other substances, such as antibiotics, it is sometimes necessary to be able to specifically treat the unborn child as well (as in the case of an ascending infection via the maternal vagina). This requires information about the concentration in which the antibiotics are transported across the placental barrier.

Most information on medication during pregnancy is based on observation and experience. Drugs are not tested on pregnant women. Fortunately! Because there are, of course, very clear ethical boundaries. Before an active substance can be administered, sufficient long-term studies must prove that it is safe to do so. Various research models such as animal experiments or studies on cell cultures are used for this purpose.

The tragic case of thalidomide illustrates what happens when drugs are not sufficiently tested before clinical use. This drug was brought onto the market without prior clinical investigation of the long-term consequences for mother and child. The active substance, thalidomide, discovered in 1954, was sold over the counter, particularly to pregnant women, as a sleep-inducing and anti-nausea agent. At the same time, an intensive advertising campaign was conducted. But as a result, thousands of children were born with severe deformities. A pharmaceutical scandal!

An overview of the use of medication during pregnancy can be found at www.embryotox.de. This is an advice center of the Charité-Universitätsmedizin Berlin, which offers free independent information on the tolerability of medicines during pregnancy and breastfeeding.

But back to placenta research: In addition to using the entire organ, only tiny parts or isolated placental cells can also be used for experiments. In toxicology experiments, for example, the effect of heavy metals on these cells is investigated. Chemotherapeutic agents used to treat maternal cancer during pregnancy are also tested on placental cells. This provides evidence of possible damage to the placental metabolism and effects on the vitality and growth of the placenta.

Another field of research is the bidirectional cell exchange between mother and child via the placenta. It is still very little studied, but fascinating. Maternal and child cells, which differ in their genetics, can implant themselves in each other's tissue and survive there for decades. This process of foreign cells surviving in the body is also known as microchimerism. A chimera is a hybrid being and the phenomenon of microchimerism refers to the smallest unit of the organism, the cell. It is divided into two types: fetal (where the child's cells are found in the mother's body) and maternal (where the mother's cells are found in the child's body). This phenomenon is currently the subject of intensive research: How does microchimerism develop? Does it have a protective or pathogenic function? However, one thing is already clear: every mother has not only an emotional, but also a lifelong cellular connection to both her own mother and her child or children.

Pregnancy-related diseases affecting the mother are another major area of research, as these also impact both the development and function of the placenta. An inadequately functioning placenta understandably affects the growth, development and sometimes even the survival of the child. In addition to pre-eclampsia, lifestyle-related diseases such as high blood pressure and diabetes in particular have been on the rise among pregnant women in recent years and are therefore increasingly becoming the subject of research.

And then of course – last but not least – there is the small and quite unusual field of research into placentophagy. There are only about a dozen scientists around the world working on this. And we can claim to be two of their number …

Basic research in the placent lab

Before we could start with the exciting experiments, we reflected on a range of preliminary considerations regarding the placentophagy project. We had to decide in advance which research questions we could formulate and which measurements we could use to answer them. And yes: there it is again, breaking down a whole world (in this case the puerperium [this is the crucial period of around six weeks after giving birth]) to a few measurable parameters. In our case, we had to translate the effects that women describe after placenta ingestion into hormones whose modes of action may be responsible for them. Our results are only one jigsaw puzzle piece of the big picture. To make our considerations comprehensible, we would therefore now like to present the postpartum period and its possible problems.

Hormone withdrawal in the puerperium

We have already presented this hypothesis in the chapter *The postnatal hormone deprivation hypothesis:* The placenta produces hormones on a partially exponential scale, which influence milk production, stress processing and social behavior. With the birth of the placenta, this "hormone factory" is lost from one day to the next, resulting in a rapid drop in hormones in the mother's blood. Some women notice this more, some women less. Of course, mothers experience a rush of feelings and emotions after the birth. The experience needs to be mentally processed. A few tears of joy or even exhaustion and overwhelm shortly after the birth are normal. However, some women want to stabilize themselves in this special situation with the help of the placenta. Surveys on placentophagy have revealed the subjective effects noticed by users: increased milk production, more energy in the postpartum period, faster recovery and a more stable mood.

Are the ingredients of the placenta responsible for these effects?

... when the mother has the blues

There are days after the birth when the mother feels exhausted. "Feeling blue": The world is crying and everything is annoying. If this state lasts a few days, goes away on its own and doesn't require any further therapeutic help, it is "only" the so-called baby blues. This is normal in the first few days after the birth and does not need to be treated. As a result of the severe hormone withdrawal, with an aching body and sore breasts, after sleepless nights, this reaction is absolutely understandable. But sometimes the sadness doesn't go away ...

Postpartum depression

Postpartum depression is a special form of the multifaceted illness of deep sadness. In the first three months after giving birth, around 20% of women develop symptoms of depression. Some mood symptoms begin during pregnancy, others start only weeks or months after the birth. A distinction is also made between the intensity or severity of the depression and its duration. And, of course, depression must be seen in context: Mothers who suffer from severe postpartum depression often have little support in puerperium. It is therefore understandable that women in this situation try everything to stabilize themselves emotionally: The reason for placentophagy in over 70% of cases is to avoid postpartum depression.

One hormone that is used for the treatment of postpartum depression is progesterone. We have therefore included it in our analysis. We also examined two neurohormones (ACTH and CRH) that influence the body's reaction to stress.

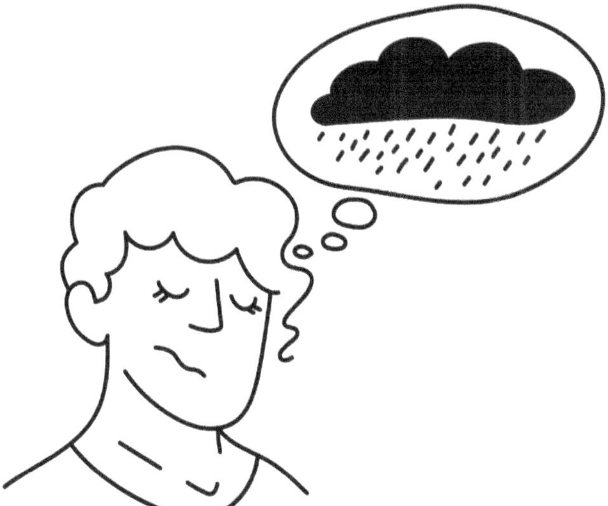

... when things aren't quite so rosy

The illness of depression has now made it into the media and social dialog, and the field of "maternal depression after childbirth" is also being increasingly researched. However, sufferers are still stigmatized or not even recognized as such. They often fall through the cracks and do not receive sufficient support. Dealing with mental illness in everyday life is a real challenge and even when correctly diagnosed, there is often a lack of treatment available. Risk factors for postpartum depression are previous depression and depressive illnesses in the family, rapid pregnancy or birth succession, many births (often more than five) and a low educational status. In addition, a non-supportive partner in the postpartum period favors maternal depression. And maternal depression in turn promotes paternal depression, i.e. depression in the father. When both parents are emotionally devastated, this is known as "parental depression" – both parents are sad, anxious, unable to care for and raise the baby, the parent-child bond suffers, and both child and parents become even sicker ... You don't need to cite any studies to understand that this initial situation is critical for children and that they can suffer from poor health for years to come. Our current social problem is that there is no screening for parental depression, and it is consequently under-diagnosed and under-treated. Conversely, this means that if we want to enable a young generation to lead a healthy life in which they can grow up strengthened by loving relationships, then we must take care of women in the postpartum period and their caregivers! The puerperium needs a lobby! Care work needs a lobby ... and postpartum depression even more so!

Some thoughts on breastfeeding

We know from traditional sources that placenta remedies were also used to promote milk production, among other things. From nature's point of view, breastfeeding is the simplest, healthiest and cheapest form of nutrition. In addition to the child, who experiences affection, love, closeness, satiety, oxytocin, security and contentment through breastfeeding, it is also good for the mother. The immediate consequence of breastfeeding is a rapid involution (shrinkage) of the uterus. Natural oxytocin is released when the baby sucks on the breast. It not only triggers the milk let-down reflex, but also causes the uterus to contract. In the first few days after giving birth some women feel the uterine contractions in their lower abdomen or in the small of the back while breastfeeding. This perception proves that newborn's suckling is successful and that the body is actively returning to its pre-pregnant state.

Another effect of breastfeeding can be weight loss. The production of breast milk is extremely strenuous, exhausting physical work that burns calories. This is why women are often so tired when breastfeeding. Not only because of the lack of sleep at night ...

Of course, milk production also requires food from which the body can filter out the essence, the best for the "liquid gold": Nuts, potatoes, lots of fresh or steamed vegetables, water, fruit plates with banana and dried fruit ... The purity and naturalness of food is the basis for the composition of breast milk. The body is constantly producing breast milk, which is always a little different, with slight variations in taste, depending on what the mother eats. This is why children who are breastfed try more foods later in life, as they are used to a variety of tastes right from the start.

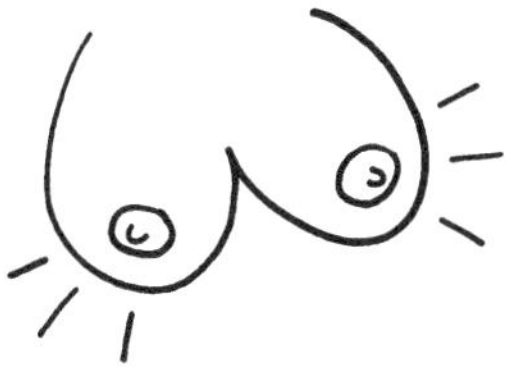

Yes, breastfeeding is not always easy, especially with the first child and at the very beginning, it requires practice, perseverance and the personal communication of tips and tricks and support from the midwife. Breastfeeding consultants can also provide helpful support in many situations. In Germany you can find good breastfeeding advice at LaLecheLiga (www.lalecheliga.de), for example.

If you have the problem of not producing enough milk as a breastfeeding mother, this can lead to real mental "stress". But which hormones are the so-called "milk boosters"? Human placental lactogen (similar in structure to the milk-forming hormone prolactin) and progesterone prepare the mother's breast for breastfeeding during pregnancy. Therefore, in addition to oxytocin, we have also included human placental lactogen in our analysis. (The effect of the hormones in detail is described in the chapter *The placenta as a hormone factory*).

The experiments begin ...

After researching the literature on the postpartum period, we thought: how exciting! And we wanted to find out more: "What is actually contained in placental tissue?" To answer this question, we needed experiments from basic research. We wanted to analyze placental tissue and examine it for selected hormones, trace elements and microorganisms. In this way, we hoped to be able to assess the benefits and possible risks of placentophagy on a scientific basis. But first we needed funding.

How can you implement your own research projects if you don't have the money? Financing smaller projects is often a major hurdle. One solution: scientific crowdfunding. With *www.experiment.com*, we opted for an English-language platform in order to achieve an international reach for our project. And it worked! We successfully raised the necessary funds and were even able to carry out a follow-up project. We would therefore like to motivate other scientists to use this opportunity to finance and implement their own projects independently of industry or other interest groups.

Thanks to the donations from the crowdfunding, the financing of our project was secured.

Before starting the experiments, we invited a specialist: Lynnea Arnold (formerly Shrief) founded IPEN (Individual Placenta Encapsulation Network) in the UK in 2010, a network that offers placenta processing services and trains "placenta encapsulation specialists".

Lynnea showed us how to process a placenta into capsules - just as mothers or placenta encapsulation specialists do at home. Because we wanted specifically to investigate what is contained in a placenta that has been processed under these real-life circumstances and not under sterile laboratory conditions.

Of course, we needed placentas for further research. These were donated to the placenta lab (Department of Obstetrics at the University Hospital in Jena) by postpartum women - with permission from the ethics committee and after written informed consent from mothers. Placentas are born at any time of the day or night, just like babies. In the lab we have an "on-call service" to receive newborn placentas from the midwives. We then either processed them straight away or (sometimes completely exhausted ourselves in the middle of the night) took them to the fridge in the lab to carry out the experiments the next day.

The placentas for our study had to fulfill several criteria: For better comparability, we only wanted to examine placentas from mature newborns. This meant that the child should not have been born prematurely. In addition, the birth should have taken place naturally and without the administration of artificial hormones (such as synthetic oxytocin). We were interested in the "imprint" of the maternal hormone situation during birth, which is stored in the placental tissue at the time of birth. In our preliminary considerations, we came to the conclusion that a planned caesarean section with spinal anesthesia could possibly create a completely different maternal hormone situation. Due to the anesthetic, the mother does not experience any pain during the caesarean section, so the body's own stress response does not run at full speed as with a vaginal birth. We have therefore included only placentas from spontaneous term deliveries. An analysis of the hormone concentration of placentas after caesarean section births would be an exciting topic for a follow-up project.

Cooked, dehydrated or raw?

The internet is full of cooking instructions and special recipes for preparing placenta. However, we wanted to use standardized methods for our project. We imitated the three most common processing methods in the laboratory: raw, raw/dehydrated and steamed/dehydrated.

There are some women who chew a small piece of placenta or place it in their cheek pouch directly after birth. The placenta smoothie is somewhat more popular, where a piece of raw placenta is chopped up beyond recognition and then pureed with fruit and juice to make a smoothie.

According to publications on placentophagy, the most common form of placenta intake is the capsule. And here there are two variants: Capsules containing raw dehydrated placental tissue and capsules containing steamed and then dehydrated placental tissue.

If one compares the preparation of the capsules with the relevant literature, the capsules with raw dehydrated placenta correspond to the traditional description from the *Pharmacopoeia of Württemberg* (see chapter *The Pharmacopoeia of Württemberg and other old medical books*). However, with the following exception: the placenta is no longer washed in wine before drying, as was recommended almost three hundred years ago. Today, our water is clean enough to rinse the placenta with.

The capsules with first steamed and then dehydrated placenta are said to comply with Chinese medicine and are therefore advertised by English and American placenta encapsulation providers as "TCM capsules". According to these organizations, the placenta is cooked over steam before drying. As part of this method of preparation, medicinal plants such as ginger, chili and lemon are often added to the water in the steamer. If you read the original texts of the Chinese *Materia Medica*, you will find different recipes. In the pharmacopoeia of the physician Li Shizhen, the powder of the dehydrated placenta is often mixed with Chinese medicinal herbs. Both steaming and subsequent dehydrating as well as drying alone without prior steaming or boiling are mentioned in this reference work.

After this preparatory work, we finally started the experiments in the laboratory. We worked on cleaned and disinfected work surfaces with clean (but not sterile) work utensils (stainless steel scissors and tweezers).

Each placenta was then processed in exactly the same way: First, we took a swab from the maternal and fetal side of the placenta to analyze the bacteria. After thorough washing with cold water, we collected general data on the placenta, namely weight, diameter and thickness. Then we divided it into three parts: one part for the analysis of raw tissue, a second part for the analysis of steamed tissue, which was then dehydrated for 12 hours at 55 degrees, and a third part for the analysis of raw dehydrated tissue, which was also dehydrated for 12 hours at 55 degrees. We wanted to find out how the concentration of the ingredients of one placenta changes as a result of steaming or dehydrating.

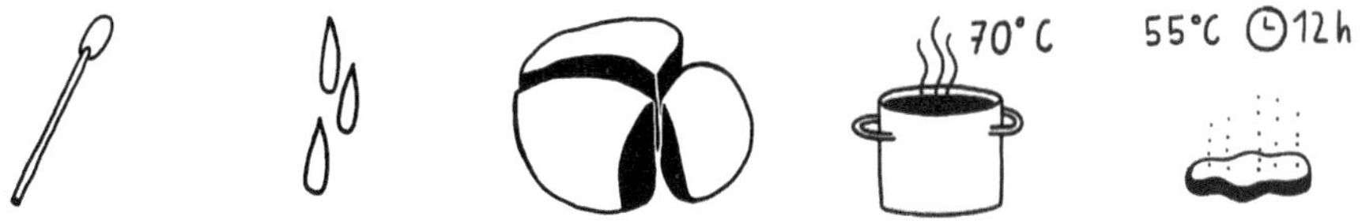

The first "raw" part of the placenta was chopped in an ordinary food processor - or to put it more correctly: "homogenized". After about 30 seconds, the tissue was finely chopped and could have been mistaken for strawberry puree. We took the samples of raw placental tissue from this "puree".

The second piece of the placenta was steamed: we placed it in a basket made of aluminum foil and cooked it in a steamer for 10 to 15 minutes. We used a meat thermometer to check that the temperature inside the piece was 70 degrees and pressed on the placenta with a fork to see if it was still bloody. When it was properly cooked, it was placed on a stainless-steel plate to cool and then cut into 0.5 centimeter thin slices. (Incidentally, this was the moment when other colleagues in the lab sniffed and tore open the windows. The steamed placenta has a very intense smell, a bit like cooking liver).

We also cut the third piece of the placenta into 0.5-centimetre-thin slices and then patted it dry with kitchen paper. Both the raw and steamed placenta strips were then dehydrated: We placed them on baking paper in a food dehydrator (a standard model used for dehydrating fruit). The strips dried for twelve hours at 55 degrees. We then subjected them to the "snap test": If you could easily break the completely dehydrated pieces, the test was successful. If the tissue was still somewhat pliable, it was dehydrated for a further two hours.

We then chopped up the dehydrated strips with the food processor and took samples for further analysis. We now had powder from raw/dehydrated tissue and steamed/dehydrated tissue. We only saved ourselves the trouble of filling the powder into capsules, as this process does not involve a concentration-changing heat application. And without a filling device, it is also hard, tedious work.

Then our sample collection was complete. We had three samples from each placenta, prepared in three different ways. These samples were all stored for a couple of weeks in the freezer of the placenta lab. Now there was only one difficulty: the analysis. The laboratory at Jena University Hospital can determine hormones, but only in blood or other body fluids such as urine. Measuring hormones in raw tissue or dried placenta powder is much more diffi- cult.

So we initiated a cooperation with a laboratory for food analysis and the biologist Ulrike Sammer. Under her supervision, the samples were processed using methods adapted specifically for our project, and the various ingredients were measured. A real challenge. To measure the steroid hormones progesterone and estrogen, the yeast receptor test used by the laboratory had to be specially adapted to our samples from placental tissue. Each hormone has a corresponding receptor that receives the hormone's information on the cell surface. The yeast receptor test not only measures the quantity of the hormone, but also whether it releases its information to the very specific receptor on the cell and activates it. As a result, we obtained an equivalent for progesterone and estrogens, i.e. not only the measured quantity of the hormones, but also an indication of their activity.

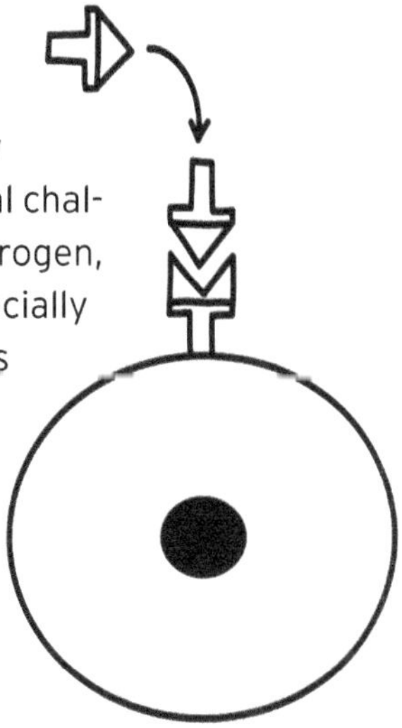

The laboratory team and we were delighted with the results! Firstly, we didn't know beforehand whether there were any measurable hormone concentrations in our samples. And secondly, none of us had expected the effects of processing to be so clearly visible.

So what's inside?

We examined six placentas, processed them in three different ways and measured six different hormones in the samples. This was possible within the budget we had acquired. To summarize our results: every placenta is a black box. It is impossible to predict what exactly is inside. The concentration of hormones and other substances varies from placenta to placenta, because it depends on the mother, her health, the birthing situation and the type of birth, the medication taken, the place of residence, lifestyle habits and so on and so forth ... Nevertheless, we were able to detect all the selected hormones in the placental tissue: CRH, ACTH, oxytocin, human placental lactogen, estrogens and progesterone.

One special thing is that these are all endogenous hormones and therefore activate exactly the corresponding receptors in the female body. They are also known as bioidentical hormones. There are small differences in the chemical structure of synthetically produced hormones.

The placentas we analyzed had an average water content of 85%. The powder, on the other hand, had – after dehydration – no water content. In order to compare dried and raw placental tissue, we therefore had to calculate the "theoretical dry weight" of raw placenta – a value that is essential for comparison. This clearly showed that most hormones are denatured – i.e. rendered useless – by heat processing.

We were the first researchers worldwide to prove that the concentration of CRH, ACTH, oxytocin, human placental lactogen and estrogens is significantly reduced by steaming and dehydration. The raw/dehydrated tissue contained significantly more hormones than the steamed/dehydrated tissue. The so-called "TCM capsules" with steamed/dehydrated tissue therefore no longer contains many hormones. The concentration of hormones was actually highest in the raw tissue. The changes in hormone concentrations due to heat processing were so significant that our results are meaningful despite the small number of cases.

However, progesterone is an exception. We had not expected that! Progesterone is the only hormone that actually increases in concentration in dehydrated tissue. Like estrogen, it is a steroid hormone. Estrogens are obviously sensitive to dehydration at 55 degrees, whereas progesterone is not. Due to the loss of water through the drying process, its relative concentration actually increases, so that the dehydrated tissue contains more progesterone than the raw tissue. Even though we were able to measure that progesterone is present in the placenta powder, we can only speculate as to whether it acts in the maternal organism after absorption via the mouth and mucous membranes or the gastrointestinal tract. In any case, it is a hormone with an important function for the maternal mood after birth, as we will look at in more detail below.

Concentrations of hormones in placental tissue

The following pages show the mean values +- standard deviation of the measured concentrations of hormones in placental tissue depending on (heat) processing.

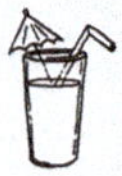

Results of the raw samples (theoretical dry weight, corresponds to 100%)

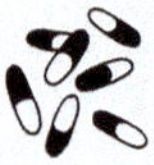

Results of the raw/dehydrated samples with indication of the concentration reduction in % of the theoretical dry weight

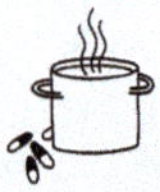

Results of the steamed/dehydrated samples with indication of the concentration reduction in % of the theoretical dry weight

Due to the wide range of detected hormone concentrations, different units are used:

pg - picogram
µg - microgram
ng - nanogram
mg - milligram

An overview of the characteristics of the different hormones can be found on p. 34-36 in the section "At a glance: important hormones produced by the placenta".

Results of the analysis of neurohormones: CRH and ACTH regulate the stress adaptation of the maternal organism.

CRH

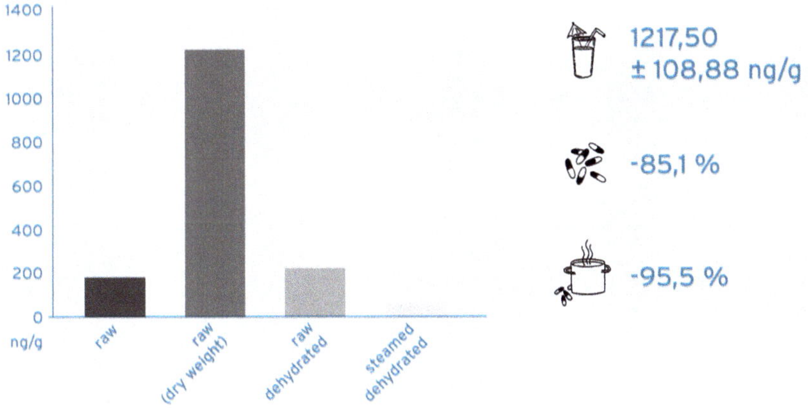

ACTH

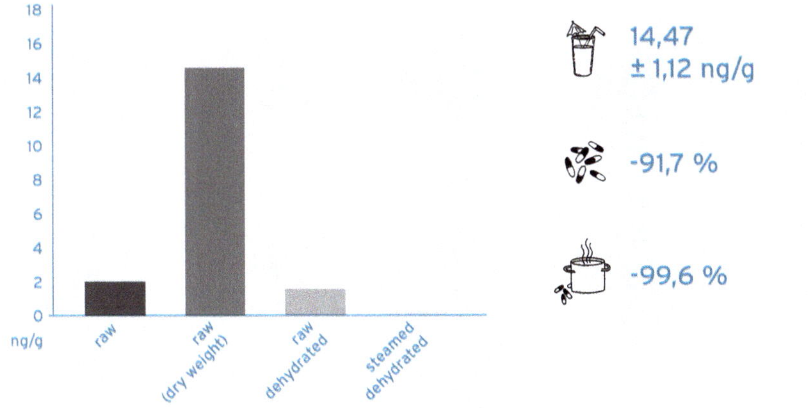

Significance for breastfeeding: The placental lactogen is contained in the milligram range in one gram of placenta tissue. Oxytocin is not quite as sensitive to dehydration.

Oxytocin

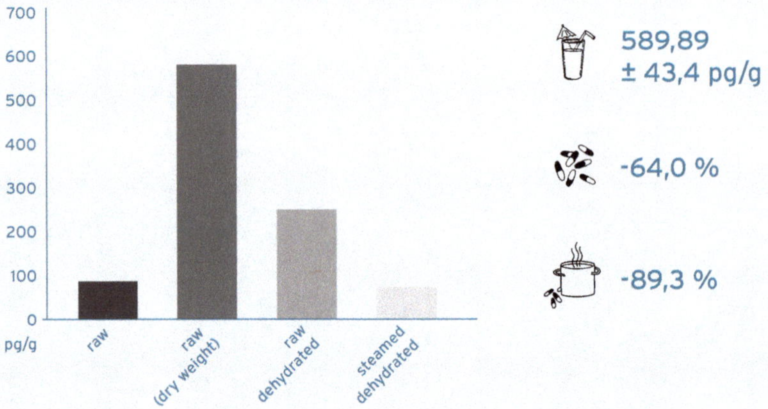

hPL

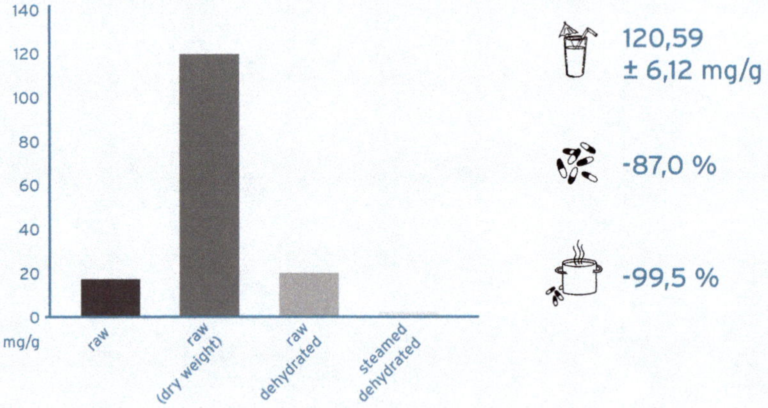

Results of the analysis of steroid hormones: Estrogens are almost completely destroyed by heat processing (steaming and dehydration) (concentration loss of 99.2%). Only progesterone is retained after drying.

Estrogen-Equivalent

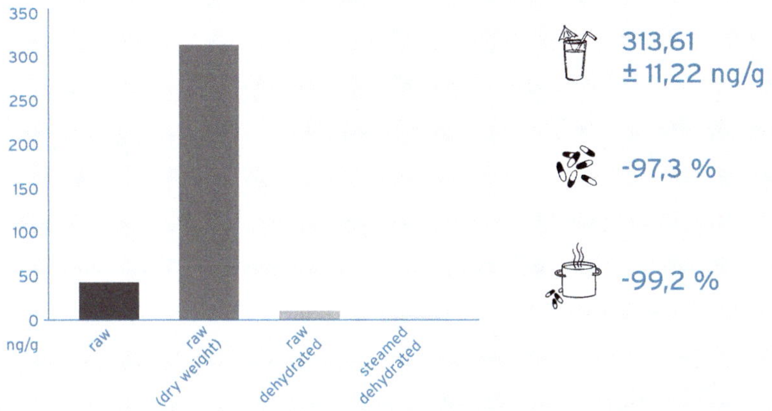

Progesterone-Equivalent

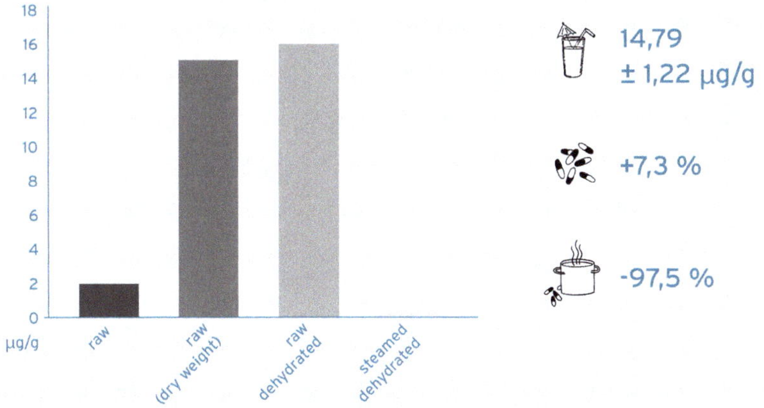

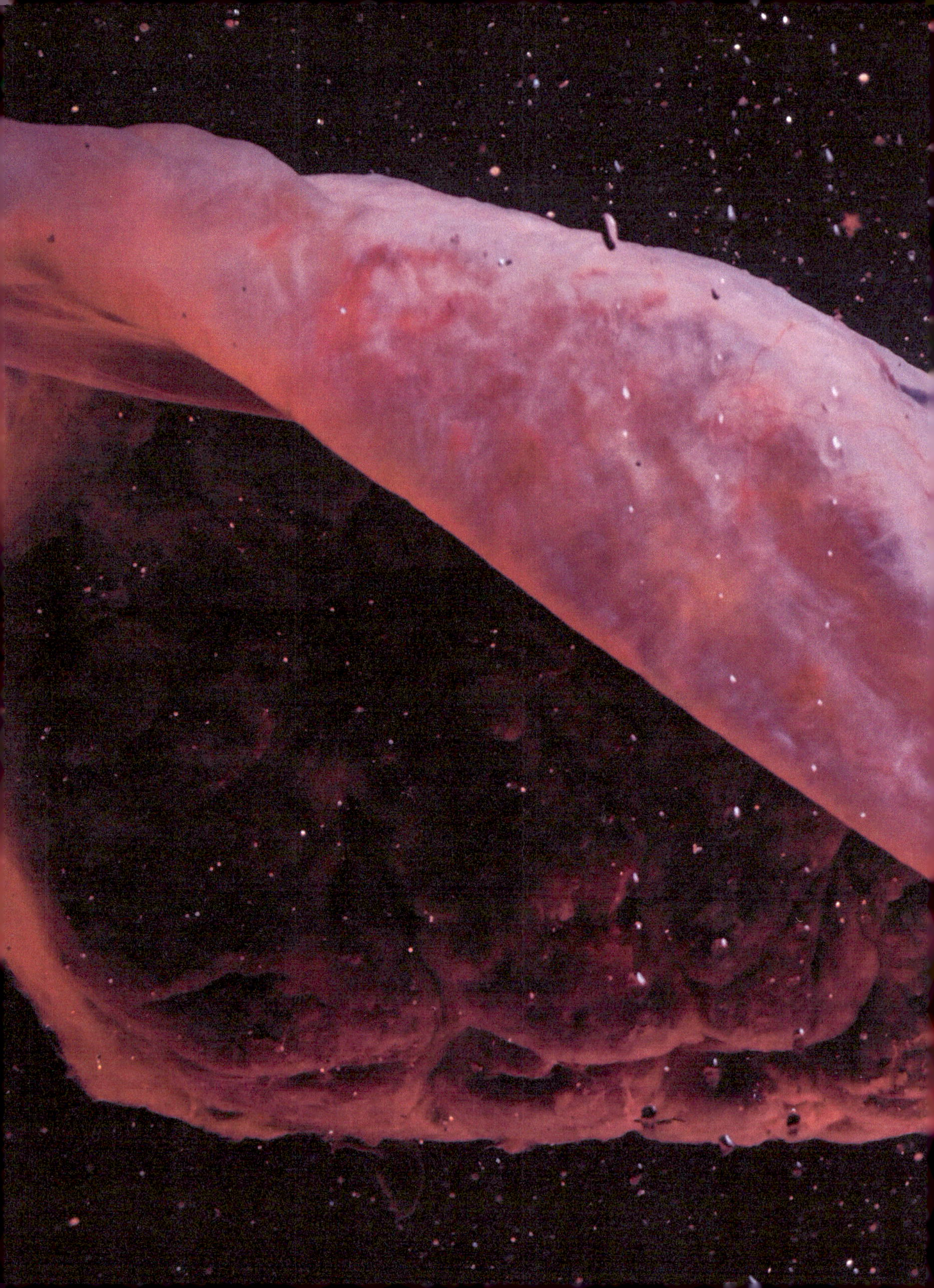

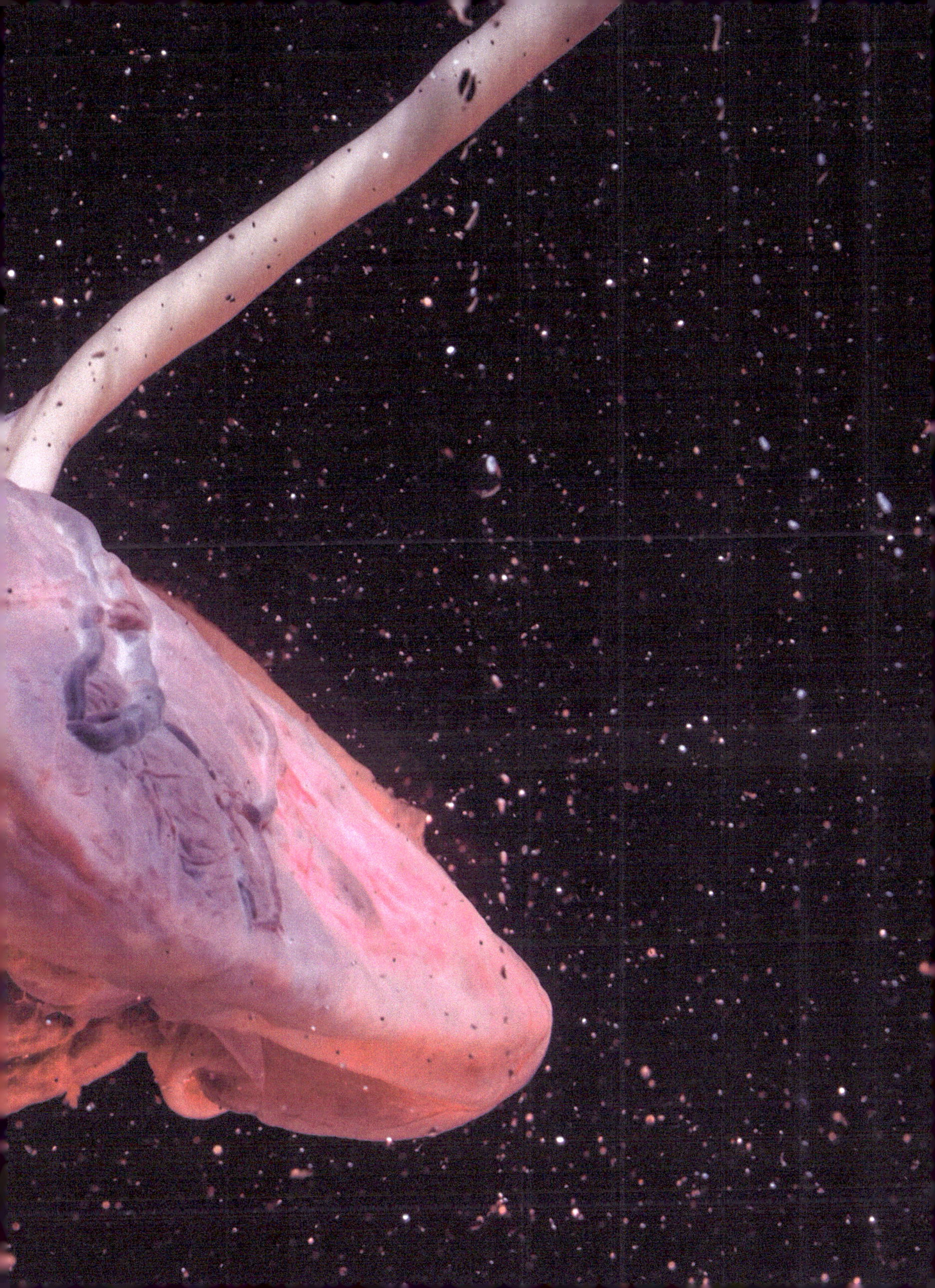

Progesterone and allopregnanolone – the female mood hormones?

We became aware of the importance of progesterone through the book *Depression after Childbirth* by Katharina Dalton. In the 1960s, this doctor was one of the first in the UK to publicly address the issue of postpartum depression. She drew parallels between premenstrual syndrome (PMS) and postpartum depression. In both cases, mood changes, exhaustion and lethargy predominate. What both disorders have in common is a noticeable drop in the blood concentration of progesterone.

In clinical studies published between 1985 and 1989, Dalton showed that 90% of women who had already suffered from depression benefited from treatment with progesterone in the event of recurrent postpartum depression. Dalton also argues that the ability to breastfeed is enhanced by the administration of progesterone. Unfortunately, however, synthetically produced progesterone is very poorly absorbed via the gastrointestinal tract. For this reason, it was given in particularly high doses as an injection into the muscle or administered as vaginal suppositories.

But perhaps – as we now suspect – it is not necessarily about the hormone progesterone itself, but about the nature and number of receptors for this hormone. You can imagine it like this: What are you supposed to do with 10,000 keys (in this case the hormone progesterone) if there is not a single lock (receptor on the cell that receives the information) for it?

As already described: Progesterone is also found in placental tissue. And its concentration is even higher after dehydration than before (while other hormones clearly lose concentration). Is there perhaps a connection between the body's own progesterone and the described "stable mood" after placenta ingestion?

Of course, it is also exciting for the pharmaceutical industry to find out how and with which medications women can be treated after giving birth. And this is where allopregnanolone comes into play. It is structurally related to progesterone. The synthetically produced allopregnanolone is also known as a "neurosteroid", as it has an effect on the brain, i.e. the regulatory circuits of the nerves. In a US study from 2018, women who suffered from postpartum depression in the first six months after giving birth were given a continuous infusion of this hormone for 60 hours. Some of them felt significantly better after the infusion, as measured on a depression scale. However, one of the most common adverse effects was "sedation", i.e. a strong drowsiness that led to a semi-conscious state.

Some things have not yet been sufficiently researched with regard to allopregnanolone: for example, it is not known what effect this high hormone dose has on the mother's hormone balance in the long-term – or on the breastfed child. Nevertheless, this study shows that the administration of the synthetic progesterone-like hormone has a clear effect on women's mood. It would be interesting to know how much natural allopregnanolone the placenta contains and whether this, like progesterone, survives the preparation process relatively unscathed. Future studies will certainly be able to provide us with answers to this question.

And (regardless of the pharmaceutical therapy) it is important to know: Mere sleep deprivation is also a risk factor for postpartum depression. If mothers can get a good night's sleep, that helps, too!

FIELD REPORT BY SELMA

I have a nineteen-year-old son and a one-year-old daughter. Nineteen years ago I was not aware of the use of the placenta in any form. Now, after learning a lot about the effects of placenta from a friend, I couldn't just throw this wonderful natural resource in the bin.

I drank a smoothie four times after the birth, spread over about four weeks. This consisted of a coin-sized piece of raw placenta mixed with fruit, yogurt and a little oil. I froze the larger part of the placenta and only processed it into powder about three months after the birth. The raw placenta is easy to process when frozen, as it can be cut into very thin slices with a sharp knife and therefore dries very quickly. I did this in the food dehydrator and it was very quick and uncomplicated. I pulverized the tissue and filled the powder into capsules.

Since then, I've always taken the encapsulated placenta when I'm not feeling so well and/or when I'm stressed, just as I feel I need them. Sometimes several days in a row, sometimes not at all for one or two weeks. I notice the effect of the placenta most clearly and almost immediately in my milk production. My daughter is now thirteen months old and I still breastfeed in the evening and at night. If I take two to three capsules a day, I notice that my breasts are heavier in the evening.

We have had very turbulent months as a couple so far and I have experienced very stressful situations and I can't say exactly what effect taking the placenta has had on my mental state, as I was still taking supplements and Schuessler cell tissue salts. But I also don't know how I would have fared if I hadn't taken the placenta capsules.

But perhaps one more comment on the effect on the psyche: after the birth of my first son, I felt very exhausted for several weeks with strong depressive traits and I was actually very worried that I would experience this again because it was terrible. But after the second birth, I didn't actually have any symptoms of total exhaustion, listlessness or sadness at all, even though the circumstances after the birth were significantly more stressful and demanding for me this time.

Trace elements in placental tissue

Nutrition Facts

Serving Size 1 Placenta (450g)

Amount Per Serving

Calories 234	Calories from Fat 33
	% Daily Values*
Total Fat 4g	**6%**
Saturated Fat 3g	**15%**
Trans Fat 0g	
Cholesterol 899mg	**300%**
Sodium 513mg	**21%**
Total Carbohydrate 2g	**1%**
Dietary Fiber 0g	**0%**
Sugars 0g	
Protein 48g	**96%**

Vitamin A 3%	Calcium 55%
Iron 149%	Selenium 127%

*Percent Daily Values are based on a 2,000 calorie diet. Your Daily Values may be higher or lower depending on your calorie needs.

	Calories	2,000	2,500
Total Fat	Less than	65g	80g
Sat Fat	Less than	20g	25g
Cholesterol	Less than	300mg	300mg
Sodium	Less than	2400mg	2400mg
Total Carbohydrate		300g	375g
Dietary Fiber		25g	30g

Funny to us is the idea from scientist Sydney Chang and her team, to depict ingredients from a human placenta on a nutrition table for food. The only thing, that would probably be unrealistic in this, is the portion size: A woman would probably rarely take in a whole placenta in one piece.

In addition to analyzing the hormones, we wanted to know whether the ingredients of the placenta pose a risk to consumers. And this is where the trace elements come into focus: The placenta does indeed contain many of them. Some of these trace elements are heavy metals. A distinction is made between trace elements that are essential for the organism (e.g. selenium) and heavy metals (e.g. iron) and non-essential, often potentially toxic heavy metals such as arsenic, lead, cadmium and mercury. For most of them, the dosage determines its level of toxicity.

Could you intoxicate yourself with placenta? Well, that will be difficult ... because we have measured the potentially harmful heavy metals and these are only contained in very small doses. If you compare these values with the maximum permitted levels for foodstuffs, then more arsenic is permitted in rice cakes for babies than can be found in raw or dehydrated placenta. Lead, arsenic, cadmium and mercury are therefore not a danger when ingesting placenta. Our results here are consistent with those of other studies.

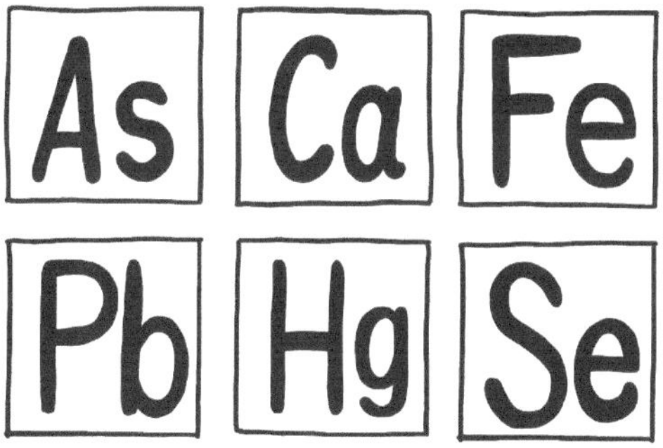

Concentrations measured in placental tissue and maximum permissible concentrations in food supplements from the European Union Food Regulation. The mean value and range (minimal to maximal concentration) are given.

	Arsenic µg/kg	**Cadmium** µg/kg	**Mercury** µg/kg
raw	5.0 (5.0-5.0)	3.0 (2.7-9.7)	1.0 (1.0-1.0)
raw/dehydrated	5.0 (5.0-16.0)	25.0 (19.0-28.0)	70.0 (3.0-99.0)
steamed/dehydrated	5.0 (5.0-14.0)	20.0 (14.0-23.0)	5.35 (3.3-19.0)
Maximum permissible concentration in food supplements	x	1000.0	100.0

	Lead µg/kg	**Selenium** µg/kg	**Iron** mg/kg
raw	26.5 (5.0-43.0)	140.0 (138.33-150.0)	84.5 (61.0-97.0)
raw/dehydrated	41.5 (18.0-250.0)	850.0 (700.0-850.0)	565.0 (450.0-600.0)
steamed/dehydrated	42.0 (15.0-220.0)	860.0 (720.0-1000.0)	475.0 (350.0-580.0)
Maximum permissible concentration in food supplements	3000.0	x	x

x means that no maximum permissible concentration is defined

Unlike in the animal world, women rarely consume their entire placenta directly after giving birth, but instead take a few capsules a day or small pieces of raw placenta. It is therefore a myth that taking placenta capsules can poison you with toxic trace elements.

Placenta is a natural source of essential trace elements such as sodium, potassium, phosphorus, calcium, copper, magnesium, zinc, selenium and iron. These are necessary for many metabolic processes. Proponents of placentophagy therefore see placenta capsules as a dietary supplement.

However, if you want to treat postpartum iron deficiency anemia, placenta will not get you very far: 20 mg of iron per day is recommended for breastfeeding women. If you take 2 capsules (500 milligrams each) of dried placenta three times a day, they contain around 1.6 milligrams of iron - this does not even cover 10% of a breastfeeding woman's daily requirement.

A brief review of the traditional use of placenta preparations: If we compare the literature of the different integrative systems of medicine, it is noticeable that a common indication for placenta use is epilepsy. We know from studies that magnesium can also be detected in dried placenta. Perhaps the historical observations on the anticonvulsant properties of placenta preparations can be explained by the effect of magnesium, the content of which can be measured in placental tissue?

Placenta as a source of energy?

Women who consume their placenta in the postpartum period report, among other things, subjectively "more energy". Could it be that a placenta smoothie is above all a good protein shake?

"Maybe you want to add some protein?" People in the US are often asked whether they want to add protein in the form of eggs or ham when they order a salad. However, in our western industrialized world, there is rarely real malnutrition. Much more frequent is obesity, which is a risk for secondary diseases of mother and child. This means that "more protein" is not generally necessary. With one exception: when breastfeeding! This is because producing milk requires a lot of energy and is a physical peak performance. Breastfeeding mothers therefore need sufficient fluids and healthy sources of energy such as nuts.

And does the mother still need placenta? Where the food shelves are overflowing, women naturally do not have to resort to their own placenta as a source of protein. A balanced and healthy diet is in such cases easily possible thanks to the constant availability of food. (By balanced and healthy, we mean home-cooked instead of ultra-processed and plastic-wrapped convenience foods). In times of scarcity, however, it is important to know that dried placenta contains a lot of protein – to be precise, placenta consists of around 80% protein.

The possibility of using placenta as an energy source was published by a Thai research team back in 2000: In a department of obstetrics, they considered that burning all placentas causes a lot of air pollution and that they could therefore be dehydrated and used as concentrated feed for animals. This would amount to an estimated 500 tons of placenta per year throughout Thailand – excluding all infectious placentas, of course. This study has given us a good overview of the trace elements and amino acids in dehydrated human placenta. But did the use as concentrated feed actually become a reality in Thailand? Unfortunately, there was nothing said about this in the publication.

Is it alive? Microorganisms in placental tissue

In addition to measuring hormones and trace elements in placental tissue, there was another important area to our research: placenta microbiology. This includes everything that is tiny and living, such as bacteria, fungi and viruses. We concentrated primarily on bacteria because we wanted to know how "alive with foreign organisms" the placenta actually is.

The very first thing we did with the newborn placentas was to take a "mibi swab" (laboratory jargon for microbiological smear). Right after birth, the placenta was swabbed from each side with a swab which looks like a cotton bud, and it is then placed in a special tube containing a solution in which microorganisms thrive. The swabs were then streaked on different agar plates (a petri dish used to culture microorganisms) on which bacteria grow. The plates with the culture medium were then placed in the incubator (nice and warm so that the organisms can multiply well) and after 48 hours we looked to see what had grown. It was quite a lot! If you want to know more, you will find a detailed overview in the appendix (see p. 170/171).

On the swabs of the maternal and fetal side of the placenta, we mainly found microorganisms that belong to the skin and vaginal flora of the woman. In other words, bacteria that are not pathogenic per se and that the body knows well. On a few occasions, we were also able to detect a fungus (*Candida albicans*) on the surface of the placenta. However, in many women this can be found in the vaginal environment without them noticing any symptoms. But if the vaginal environment gets out of balance (see chapter *The vaginal microbiome*), it can lead to an itchy fungal infection.

But what happens to the microorganisms after cleaning, steaming and dehydrating?

We were able to show that washing the placenta under running water has a significant effect and that many of these small organisms are simply rinsed away. Dehydration led to a further reduction in the number of microorganisms. There were hardly any bacteria left in the steamed/dehydrated tissue. And what happened to the fungus? After dehydration, *Candida albicans* was also no longer detectable on the placental tissue.

Impact of processing to the number of species detected.

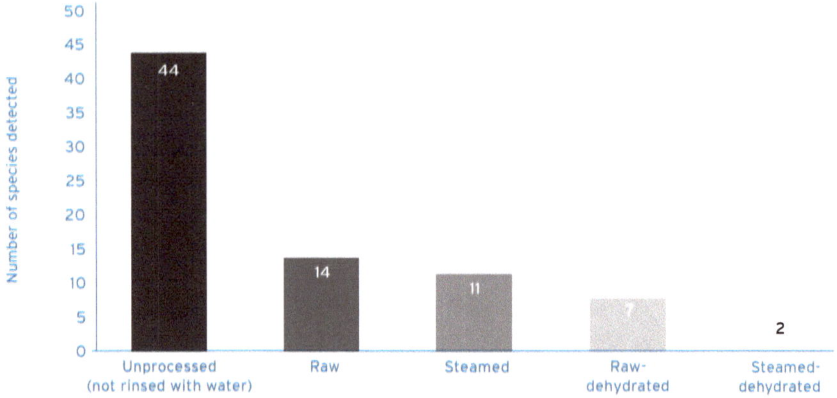

It can therefore be said that heat processing significantly reduces the microorganisms (the vast majority of which are friendly inhabitants of the female genital area). At the same time, however, the hormones the tissue contains are also destroyed. A compromise is therefore to use the raw placenta after washing it thoroughly under cold running water.

What we have not examined are viruses in placental tissue. The cultivation of living viruses is much more difficult than, for example, the detection of genetic fragments using "PCR". This "polymerase chain reaction" is a laboratory test that can detect fragments of (viral) genetic material, but it does not provide any information to whether these viruses are dead or alive.

In Germany, screening is part of prenatal care and some infections such as HIV, hepatitis B, syphilis or rubella can be excluded by means of a blood test. The urine is also tested for the bacterium *Chlamydia trachomatis*, as chlamydia can lead to an infection without any symptoms being noticed. The pregnant woman can also be tested for toxoplasmosis and the cytomegalovirus. This screening will eliminate some viral and bacterial maternal infections. However, screening can never remove all theoretically possible risks. Rare pathogens such as Zika viruses or plasmodia, which can cause malaria, are not tested for.

Microbiological digression: the group of B streptococci

There are a few bacteria to which special attention is paid in obstetrics and neonatology (the special care of newborns): Group B streptococci, Latin *Streptococcus agalactiae*. In English, "Group B Streptococci" is often abbreviated to "GBS".

B streptococci live symbiotically with other microorganisms of the gastrointestinal tract or the urogenital system. Sometimes B streptococci can also be found in the vagina without causing disease. This is referred to as colonization with B streptococci, which affects around 18% of pregnant women worldwide. Pregnant women can have a screening for B streptococci carried out between the 35th and 37th week of pregnancy. If the test result is positive, the mother is recommended antibiotic treatment during childbirth. This is because if B streptococci are transmitted to the newborn during birth, these bacteria *can* be the trigger for a serious infection in the newborn - this is known as sepsis (or colloquially "blood poisoning"). Fortunately, this early B-streptococcal sepsis is extremely rare, affecting less than one in a thousand newborns.

However, in order not to overlook the rare cases of newborn infection, midwives, pediatricians and postnatal nurses pay close attention to the children in their first days of life. Symptoms are not always obvious even to new parents, as sometimes only a sleepiness of the child, a grayish skin color or a pronounced sensitivity to touch are noticeable. However, newborns with an infection can also experience a drop in oxygen saturation in the blood - which is why pulse oximetry, i.e. the measurement of the oxygen content in the blood, is part of newborn screening in Germany. Children whose mothers have a positive B-streptococcus status according to the maternity record are regularly checked by the postnatal caregivers in the first 48 hours of life (does the child appear ill?) and the temperature and circulation of the newborn are checked.

However, not all B streptococci are the same. There are different subgroups, some of which are more aggressive, others more harmless. Perhaps we also need to change our perspective completely and ask whether streptococci are not simply easy to cultivate on the samples taken and are therefore more frequently identified as pathogens?

It is now also suspected that there is an interplay between severe neonatal infections and the child's immune system. This is because, compared to the frequency of B streptococci, severe newborn sepsis is a rarity.

But what does this microbiological digression have to do with eating placenta?

"Do not eat your placenta – you can sicken or kill your baby ..."
Really? How did this drastic warning come about?

In 2018, there was a single case published by the American health authority, the Center for Disease Control (CDC): A newborn suffered from a B Streptococcus infection after birth (early-onset sepsis) and was treated in the neonatal intensive care unit. After a few days, the infant was discharged home. Five days after discharge, the child was treated again in hospital – again with a B streptococcal infection (late-onset sepsis). As the mother had taken her placenta in the form of capsules, these were examined: The same subtype of B streptococcus as the one that caused the infant's sepsis was found in the capsules. Although the breast milk was free of B streptococci, the CDC concluded that the ingestion of the placenta capsules was the cause of the child's early and late neonatal sepsis. We also discussed the individual case in the team of the Department of Obstetrics in Jena. We came up with the following hypothesis: The mother was probably a carrier of the B streptococcus subtype before and after birth and transmitted the bacteria to the newborn through close contact with the child (kissing and cuddling). However, we cannot prove this hypothesis.

The B streptococcus project

"Impact of tissue processing on microbiological colonization in the context of placentophagy". You can read the open access publication via this link.

Of course, we could not leave this individual case as it was, but wanted to know how dangerous it is if you want to ingest encapsulated placenta with a positive test for B streptococci in the pregnancy screening. We set up a clinical-experimental study to get to the bottom of this question.

We collected placenta donations from women who tested positive for B streptococcus according to their maternity records. When a woman came to the delivery room to give birth, we took another vaginal and rectal swab for B streptococci to confirm the colonization. This is because a positive B streptococcus test at 36 weeks of pregnancy does not necessarily mean that it will also be positive at the time of birth. This was also shown by our results: Out of 17 women who tested positive for B streptococcus according to their maternity passports, we were able to confirm the streptococcus finding in 12 cases, all others were negative.

After birth, we processed and examined the placentas in the same way as in the first series of experiments. Exception: We only dried the placenta pieces for eight hours (instead of 12 previously) because we wanted to know whether a shorter dehydration time would also effectively remove microorganisms.

We also wanted to answer the following question: If women had a positive smear test for B streptococci in the vagina or rectal region during pregnancy, can B streptococci be detected on the placenta after birth?

Our result was: B streptococci are rarely found on placenta surface after birth. These bacteria can be transferred from the mother's vaginal area to the placental surface during a caesarean section as well as during a vaginal birth. In our study, B streptococci were only found on the surface of two out of thirteen placentas (corresponding to 15 %) in women testing positive for B streptococci. This is probably due to the administration of the antibiotic ampicillin during childbirth. Likewise, one of seven women who were not screened for B streptococci was an asymptomatic carrier of B streptococci in the pre-birth smear. The bacteria were then no longer detectable on the placenta.

We also wanted to know: Can B streptococci be found on processed placenta? The answer: no! Rinsing the placenta thoroughly under cold running water after birth removes many microorganisms, including B streptococci. Heat processing like steaming and dehydrating (at 54 degrees Celsius) also significantly reduces the number of B streptococci, as the bacteria are very sensitive to high temperatures. In our clinical study both types of pulverized placenta (raw/dehydrated and steamed/dehydrated) and also raw tissue were free of B streptococci. These results would have to be verified by a study with a larger sample size. We processed a total of 24 placentas.

Basic data and results of the GBS study
(GBS = Group B Streptococci)
The placenta samples were divided into different groups depending on the mode of birth, the GBS status of the mother and the antibiotic therapy administered.

	Birth mode	Antibiotic treatment	Placentas processed	GBS-Swab positive vaginal/rectal	GBS on placenta surface	GBS on processed samples
GBS positive according to maternity record	spontaneous	no	3	1	-	-
		Yes	10	8	1	-
	C-section	no	4	3	1	-
Screening for GBS not carried out	spontaneous	no	3	-	-	-
	C-section	no	4	1	-	-
total			24	13	2	0

To underline our results from the clinical part of the study, we added another experiment. What happens when the placenta is artificially contaminated with high doses of bacteria? We had special and particularly aggressive bacteria cultivated: B streptococci and the bacterium *Escherichia coli*, both of which are common pathogens of neonatal sepsis. We then artificially "inoculated" placentas with enormously high doses of these pathogens. These experiments also showed that processing the tissue with heat has a significant effect in reducing the number of bacteria.

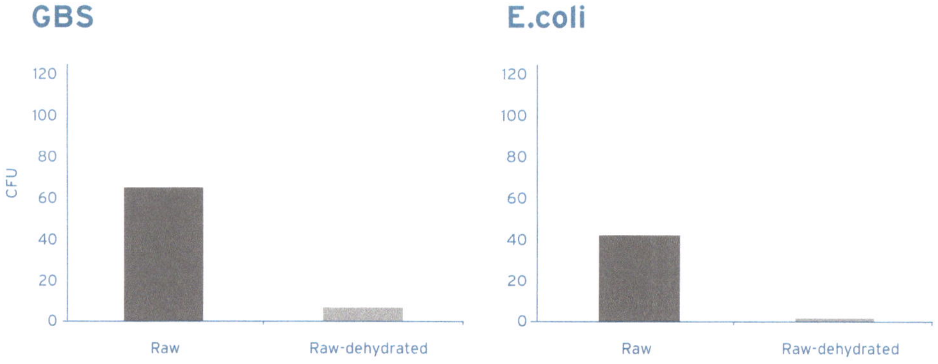

With our B streptococcus study, we were therefore able to show that very few to none of these bacteria should be found in placenta smoothies or placenta capsules. And: not all bacteria that we ingest with our food make us ill.

Fortunately, we humans have "stomach protection". With its low pH value, stomach acid is an important barrier for pathogens (unless you take stomach acid blockers like proton pump inhibitors – PPIs). Streptococci, which are ingested with food, hardly ever survive the acidic environment of the stomach. It is not always guaranteed whether the capsules for self-filling are really "gastric juice resistant" and actually only dissolve in the duodenum. A number of factors have an influence on the gastric juice resistance: the starting material (gelatin or plant-based), an additional special coating for some capsule types, the time of ingestion (time spent in the empty stomach) and other factors. Perhaps some of the B streptococci do make it into the gastrointestinal tract. But how could they get from there into breast milk? For B streptococci to get into breast milk, you would have to have a lot of bacteria in your blood (and thus be seriously ill) in order to transfer them to the newborn via the milk, which could then cause an infection.

In conclusion, one can say: "Everyone remembers the case report." The warnings circulating on the internet that eating the placenta could make the baby ill or kill it do not reflect the current state of scientific knowledge. A large data analysis of 23,242 out-of-hospital births in the USA shows that placenta ingestion does not pose an increased risk to the newborn. The risk factors examined within the first six weeks after birth are: death of the newborn, admission to a neonatal intensive care unit and admission to hospital.

Either way, a sensible risk assessment is always necessary. If mothers with a positive B-streptococcus result are unsure – they can always plant a tree over their placenta.

Microorganisms and food

How "germy" is our food actually? Can you compare animal meat with raw human placenta? How many fecal germs (such as Escherichia coli) are actually allowed in raw minced meat?
These and similar questions can be confusing at first glance. However, we have given a lot of thought to this exciting comparison. Because if placenta is classified as a food or food supplement, the European Union's food regulations would apply. These regulations stipulate, for example, that the following bacteria cannot be present in dried foods for special medical purposes: ***Listeria monocytogenes,*** Salmonella spp, Enterobacter sakazakii, Escherichia coli and Staphylococcus aureus. The placenta samples in our studies were free of these bacteria and would therefore comply with the regulation for foodstuffs.
But what about raw meat? If you go shopping for poultry in Germany, up to 59% of meat is contaminated with bacteria. These include many antibiot-

ic-resistant germs such as MRSA (methicillin-resistant *Staphylococcus aureus*) and ESBL (bacteria resistant to **β-lactam antibiotics**), which are "bred" through the uncontrolled use of antibiotics in factory farming.
So to return to the question of whether animal meat and human raw placenta can be compared: We did not find multi-resistant germs such as MRSA and ESBL on the samples of washed raw placenta.

The toxic placenta

Besides all the fascination for the natural ingenuity of the placenta as an organ, we cannot leave out an important aspect of placenta research. Unfortunately, it becomes somewhat unromantic when we talk about the placenta from a toxicological perspective. This is because toxicology deals with poisonous, potentially harmful substances.

Is the placenta, as a protective shield and filter, enriched with hazardous substances at the end of pregnancy? And what about the omnipresent environmental chemicals? Which substances can have a particularly strong influence on a developing fetus in the most sensitive phase of life? What can the placenta filter to protect the child and what does it let through?

Particularly if women are thinking about using their own placenta as a remedy, we cannot leave out this area of placenta research and would like to give an insight into the topic of toxicology here. And first of all we have to say (as is so often the case in science): There is still a lot we don't know. Given the wide range of chemicals used by mankind, toxicology is a huge field of research that will keep us busy in the future.

Environmental toxins

Unfortunately, environmental toxins surround us constantly and everywhere. Contact with them can hardly be avoided. And the fetus is also exposed to them in the particularly sensitive phase of development and maturation.

Environmental toxins include pesticides, persistent organic pollutants (POPs), plastics and their by-products, phyto- and mycoestrogens and toxins, by-products from heating and curing food, pollutants from traffic and industry and metals. Environmental toxins can influence or even reinforce each other. Many of these chemicals show placental transfer, and even if they do not cross the placental barrier, or only to a small extent or very slowly, some of them have an influence on the function and metabolism of the placenta itself and thus, of course, indirectly on the unborn child.

Nanoparticles, i.e. tiny particles in the nanometer range that are produced industrially or unintentionally through degradation or combustion processes, can also cause direct or indirect harm to the fetus. Industrially produced nanoparticles can be found in a variety of foods, paints, varnishes, medicines and cosmetics. Titanium dioxide particles (E171) led to altered placental anatomy in rats - and can be found everywhere, whether as a "whitener" in toothpaste or sunscreen, or in medicines such as ibuprofen. Until mid-2022, E171 was also found in many foods and sweets. It was found in mozzarella, mayonnaise, marshmallows - and many other foods. Following a new risk assessment, a mutagenic effect could no longer be ruled out and the European Union banned titanium dioxide as an additive in food.

Particulate matter

Other environmental toxins are produced when diesel is burned. Black soot particles, components of particulate matter, accumulate in the placenta and have also been detected on the fetal side of the human placenta. The higher the mother's exposure to particulate matter at her place of residence, for example if she lives in a large city, near an industrial site or on a busy road, the higher the concentration in the placenta.

Frequently occurring POPs (persistent organic pollutants) – poorly degradable, carbon-containing environmental pollutants

Name	Example of Usage
PFAs (per- and polyfluorinated alkyl substances)	more than 10,000 different substances; in cosmetics, cookware (Teflon®), paper coatings, textiles, ski waxes, pesticides or fire extinguishing, agents for surface treatment of metals and plastics
PCBs (polychlorinated biphenyls)	until 1986 in transformers, electrical capacitors, as sealants, hydraulic fluids and plasticizers in paints and plastics; still found in the envi ronment and food chain as well as in foodstuff due to their longevity
Dioxins and furans	Industrial by-products and incineration residues
DDT (dichlorodiphenyltri-chloroethane)	widely used insecticide until the 1970s; still found in the environment, food chain and foodstuffs due to its longevity

Microplastics

When plastic is exposed to mechanical influences or solar radiation, it breaks down into tiny particles - plastic particles in the micrometer range. Microplastics can now be found everywhere on our beautiful planet, even in uninhabited places such as the Arctic. It is therefore not surprising that these particles are also present in the human body and blood, and can cross the human placental barrier. A team led by Italian Antonio Ragusa was able to detect pigmented microplastic fragments in the size range of 5 to 10 micrometers in four out of six placentas examined, both on the mother's and the child's side. As a result, they coined the term "plasticenta".

Even smaller plastic particles of nanometer size, also known as nano plastics, are often produced industrially and can also pass through the placental barrier. And: the smaller they are, the easier they transfer from the mother to the unborn child.

It is not only the plastic particles themselves that pollute our environmental system. Plasticizers such as bisphenols and phthalates are needed for the production of plastic or resins. The best known is bisphenol A, which can leach from plastic packaging into food, has been linked to tumor growth and heart disease as well as fertility problems, and it has therefore been banned from baby bottles and pacifiers for several years. Phthalates are now banned in toys but can still be found in plastic packaging. Plasticizers and other substances such as triclosan (biocide and preservative), parabens (preservative) and substance classes such as POPs are also referred to as endocrine disruptors.

Excursus: endocrine disruptors

Endocrine disruptors are harmful chemicals that disrupt the body's endocrine system as they act in a similar way to the body's own hormones. More than 800 chemicals are known, and the number is rising. Disruptions occur primarily in hormone metabolism. Endocrine disruptors are suspected of causing hormone-dependent tumors, promoting obesity and diabetes and generally disrupting fertility, for example through a reduced sperm count. Many of these substances influence the growth and development of the placenta and overcome the placental barrier. They have a direct negative influence on the developing fetus during its most sensitive phase of life.

To summarize: Environmental toxins are a topic that is hard to swallow! And it doesn't get any easier when you consider that our environment, groundwater and all our bodies (whether pregnant or non-pregnant, human, animal or plant) contain a well-stirred and shaken cocktail of hundreds of these substances. Nevertheless, the dosage determines their toxicity.

We can avoid plastic in general and plastic food packages in particular, we can use water filters, opt for natural cosmetics in glass bottles, consume organic food and take long walks in the forest: By doing so, we are not only doing our bit for the environment, we can also reduce our individual risk of exposure to environmental toxins.

THE STATE OF RESEARCH ON PLACENTOPHAGY

The problem with clinical research using human placenta is that this tissue poses a potential risk of infection as it is not sterile. Furthermore, placenta cannot be standardized. The composition of substances varies from woman to woman, and it is not possible to specify an exact dose of ingredients - and this is one of the reasons why so far clinical studies have failed to be feasible. Furthermore, it takes a lot of money, time and patience, to overcome the legal hurdles. But there is a clever team in Las Vegas led by Sharon Young, Laura Gryder and Daniel Benyshek who have been able to carry out randomized, placebo-controlled studies despite these difficulties.

We know from these studies that the concentration of hormones in the mother's saliva changes slightly as a result of taking the capsules. For example, a significantly higher level of 17-hydroxyprogesterone (an intermediate product in the production of sex hormones) was found in the placenta-consuming group. However, a truly resounding effect on the postpartal mental status, maternal exhaustion or bonding could not be demonstrated.

Interestingly, only "TCM capsules" were used for these studies. Our experiments in the placenta lab showed that up to 99.5% of the tissue hormones are destroyed during heat processing such as steaming and dehydrating. Maybe the studies weren´t able to show groundbreaking results because almost all hormone content in the placenta capsules was already lost through processing. It would make sense to carry out the studies again with raw placental tissue and also to investigate the effect of placenta ingestion on maternal milk production. After all, according to historical sources and reports from women, lactation stimulation is a direct effect of placenta ingestion. But perhaps it is the heat processing that makes the difference: According to the original Chinese texts, the placenta was not steamed and dehydrated in all recipes, but in many cases only dried and supplemented with medicinal herbs.

Apart from the new RCTs (randomized, controlled trials), the gold standard of clinical studies, there have been over a hundred years of research on placenta as a remedy. Although the quality and conduct of the studies can be criticized from today's perspective, the researchers at that time tried to gather new information to the best of their knowledge and belief and within the scope of their possibilities.

A historical study from 1918 describes the influence of ingestion of pulverized placenta tissue on milk production: An increased content of protein and lactose in breast milk was measured. The exclusively breastfed infants from mothers in the placenta-intake group also showed faster weight gain than those in the comparison group without placenta ingestion. And although no hormones were known at that time, it was possible to demonstrate their effects in clinical trials – using a living example.

The following outline of scientific work on placentophagy in the animal kingdom and in humans is not complete, but it provides a good overview of the historical and current issues.

Selection of publications on human placentophagy	**Results**
Hammett (1917): *The effect of the ingestion of desiccated placenta on the variations in the composition of human milk during the first eleven days after parturition*	The contained protein and lactose levels in breast milk increased after ingestion of dehydrated placenta.
Hammett (1918): *The effect of the maternal ingestion of desiccated placenta upon the rate of growth of breast-fed infants*	The exclusively breastfed infants of mothers who ingested dehydrated placenta showed a faster weight gain compared to the group without placenta intake.
Soykova-Pachnerova (1954): *Placenta as a Lactagogon*	The hormones contained in dehydrated placenta led to increased milk production in 86.2 % of women (n=181), placentophagy as a therapeutic option for hypogalactia (lack of milk production).
Selander (2013): *Human maternal placentophagy: a survey of self-reported motivations and experiences associated with placenta consumption*	Women (n=189) described the following subjective benefits after placentophagy: improved mood in the postpartum period, more energy, increased milk production, reduced bleeding and faster recovery.
Gryder (2017): *Effects of Human Maternal Placentophagy on Maternal Postpartum Iron Status: A Randomized, Double-Blind, Placebo-Controlled Pilot Study*	Placentophagy has neither a positive nor a negative effect on postpartum maternal iron status. Placenta capsules are not a sufficient therapy for postpartum anemia.
Young (2017): *Effects of placentophagy on maternal salivary hormones: A pilot trial, part 1*	The ingestion of steamed, dehydrated placenta leads to small but significant changes in the hormone profile of women.

Selection of publications on human placentophagy	**Results**
Young (2017): *Placentophagy's effects on mood, bonding, and fatigue: A pilot trial, part 2*	The ingestion of steamed, dehydrated placenta does not lead to any significant change in maternal mood, bonding and fatigue.
Young (2016): *Human placenta processed for encapsulation contains modest concentrations of 14 trace minerals and elements* Chang (2017): *Nutritional composition and heavy metal content of the human placenta* Johnson (2018): *Human placentophagy: Effects of dehydration and steaming on hormones, metals and bacteria in placental tissue*	Analysis of trace elements in placental tissue: no risk of intoxication. Potentially harmful trace elements only contained in marginal doses.
Young (2016): *Presence and concentration of 17 hormones in human placenta processed for encapsulation and consumption* Johnson (2018): *Human placentophagy: Effects of dehydration and steaming on hormones, metals and bacteria in placental tissue*	Placental tissue as a natural source of endogenous hormones. The concentration of hormones in the tissue changes significantly due to heat processing.
Benyshek (2018): *Placentophagy among women planning community births in the United States: Frequency, rationale, and associated neonatal outcomes*	Almost a third of mothers from non-clinical births take their placenta postpartum, in 73% of cases the reason is to avoid postpartum depression. There is no increased risk for the newborn due to maternal placentophagy.

Selection of publications on human placentophagy	Results
Johnson (2022): Impact of tissue processing on microbiological colonization in the context of placentophagy Johnson (2018): Human placentophagy: Effects of dehydration and steaming on hormones, metals and bacteria in placental tissue	Placental tissue primarily harbors microorganisms from the skin and vaginal flora. Heat processing significantly reduces the microorganisms. Placenta ingestion is unlikely to be a cause for infections.
Münz (2020): Placentophagie - Erfahrungen von Anwenderinnen und Entwicklung eines Informationsblattes	The intake of placenta in the postpartum period showed positive effects on milk production (90%), uterine involution (88%) and mood (82%), subjective information provided by the participants.
Johnson (2022): Placenta tissue processing protocol - in the context of placentophagy	Detailed protocol for placenta processing

Selection of publications on placentophagy (animal kingdom)	**Results**
Blank (1980): Effects of placentophagy on serum prolactin and progesterone concentrations in rats after parturition or superovulation	In rats, the ingestion of placenta led to increased serum prolactin levels and reduced serum progesterone levels compared to the non-intake group. Placenta contains substances that influence hormone levels (prolactin, progesterone) after absorption via the oral mucosa.
Schmidt (1976): Verhalten einer Zoogruppe von Halsband-Pekaris (Tayassu tajacu)	The induction of lactation ("wet-nurses") in mammals which have not experienced pregnancy by placenta ingestion combined with stimulation of the breast by sucking has been described.
Kristal (1991): Enhancement of opioid-mediated analgesia: a solution to the enigma of placentophagia	A factor is called placental opioid enhancing factor (POEF) has been investigated in rats. POEF enhances the body's own analgesia: natural painkillers produced in the brain (opioids). In addition, animals from the placentophagy group showed an accelerated onset of maternal behavior.

The shaky pillars of evidence-based medicine

by Sophia Johnson

An overview of the current state of research shows that many questions relating to placentophagy have already been scientifically investigated. In our modern society, we want "evidence" for all therapeutic activities. The desire for this is absolutely understandable and justified. Medical decisions should be made on a sound scientific basis. Nowadays, however, "evidence-based medicine" is often equated with "clinical trials". This leaves out something essential!

David Sacket was a professor at Oxford, working at the Center for Evidence-Based Medicine. He formulated the three pillars of evidence-based medicine that should be taken into account in order to be a good doctor. Treatment decisions should be based on: individual clinical expertise (i.e. the doctor's own medical experience), the best available external evidence (scientific data) and the patient's wishes.

In today's medicine, the latter is often given far too little attention. In fact, it is rarely about the patient's wishes. Treatment is based on guidelines and, above all, supposedly cost oriented – and this has led to a catastrophic situation in the German healthcare system. When health is used for capitalist purposes and doctors no longer focus on the meaning of their work because their main aim is to generate profits for a company – then something is going wrong. Health is a common good! And as much as the health sector is used to maximize profits, science has developed into an interest-based industry. (I'm glad of any exception to this dystopian scenario!)

In the publication *The Illusion of Evidence-Based Medicine*, researchers clearly describe what the problem is today: Science is intertwined with corporate interests, there are no laws to curb them, which has led to a commercialization of the scientific world.

Clearly, clinical studies are necessary if the effects of medical preparations are to be demonstrated. If the aim is to find out whether a new drug is safe, then of course clinical trials are necessary. However, they are incredibly expensive and usually very time-consuming. Where does the money come from and where can industry-independent, transparent research be found? Fundraising can be used to identify which issues have reached the mainstream of research funding – and which topics are falling by the wayside. Placentophagy is one of the latter. Therefore, with public crowdfunding, we have found a way to finance our research free from third-party interests.

Apart from the clinical studies (the external evidence), it is also important to consider the internal evidence, the experience of the doctors and therapists. In our case, there is empirical evidence – gathered through experience – for placenta as a remedy. We assume that the historical sources, some of which we have already cited, are based on the experience of doctors of the time. Another example of practical experience with placenta remedies is the statement by the 16th century Chinese physician Wu Qiu: "Placentas are used to cure men and women of all deficiency diseases, extreme states of exhaustion, at the height of serious illnesses and in epilepsy (with loss of mind and unconsciousness). Placentas calm the heart and nourish the blood. They strengthen the Qi and replenish the essence."

These therapeutic experiences were made at a time when neither blood analyses, ultrasound nor other diagnostic examinations other than one's own perception could be used. Are they therefore less valid because they cannot be measured and standardized in the sense of today's clinical studies?

Apart from internal and external evidence, however, we should first and foremost turn our attention to the patients: The women after childbirth and their individual wishes for medical treatment.

We love questioning science!

There are women who want a self-determined birth - if possible, without external interventions. There are also women who would like to give birth out of hospital, i.e. at home or in a birthing center. We know from American data that women who do not give birth in a clinical setting often use their placenta as a remedy in the postpartum period.

The German Society for Quality in Out-of-Hospital Birth (QUAG) exists to assess the safety of these births in Germany. The aim of QUAG is to make the quality of obstetric care provided by midwives in birth centers or at home births visible. Data surrounding the birth is collected and is then available for analyses, scientific evaluations and publications.

In the US, the benefits and risks of out-of-hospital birth are examined in scientific discussions, too; always with a view to the safety of mother and child. However, we sometimes observe a tendency to confirm prejudices in these publications.

For example, in the publication *Alternative Birth Plans and Unintended Maternal and Neonatal Consequences: A Review of the Literature*, the authors claimed that heavy metals such as cadmium, lead and mercury accumulated in the placenta and concentrations of heavy metals in placenta capsules reached or exceeded the limits for foodstuffs. The authors concluded that placentophagy should be avoided due to risks and lack of benefits, and that women who wish to ingest their placenta should be advised not to do so. Unfortunately, in this section of the publication, the data was skewed. Our study (and other scientific publications) showed exactly the opposite: potentially toxic trace elements are only marginally present in placental tissue and are well below the permitted level for food (see chapter ***Trace** elements in placental tissue*).

One might think that the intention to judge alternative birth practices as risky and potentially infectious can be read from the discussion and preparation of the data. It does not seem as if the authors were objective in their assessment of the literature.

In any case, it makes sense to make a critical risk-benefit assessment based on scientific data. However, interpreting data in a way that suits the opinion of the authors is contrary to good scientific practice.

In a similar way to the report in this scientific publication, the facts were also misrepresented in a popular science report on "Placenta in the oven" by the German newspaper *SPIEGEL*. Allegedly, "masses" of estrogens are still present in the placenta tissue after drying. However, our experiments have also shown that these hormones lose 99% of their concentration during steaming and drying.

Even if you google "should I eat my placenta" (as we did on February 28, 2023), the search engine gives us the following answer as a highlighted snippet: "… there's no evidence that eating the placenta provides health benefits. Placentophagy can be harmful to you and your baby." However, this statement contradicts the scientific data: a 2018 study of 23,242 women in the USA found that placenta ingestion poses no increased risk to the child (hospital admission, treatment in intensive care, infant death within the first six weeks of life) or to the woman. Why does this warning appear so prominently in the search engine algorithm? Does this mainly refer to the single case of B streptococcal infection of a newborn (see chapter *Microbiological digression: the group of B streptococci*)? Here, too, we unfortunately have to conclude that this information does not correspond to the current state of research.

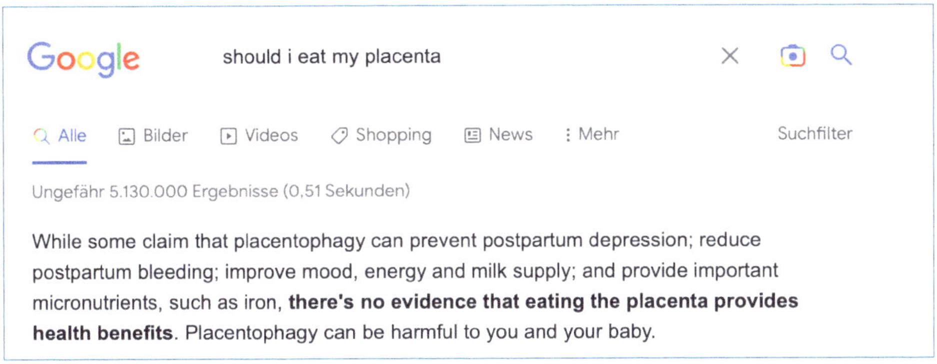

A search query on February 28, 2023 at www.google.de

If you type in your search engine the German keywords "Plazenta essen" (ingesting placenta), the answer is different: Subjective effects of placentophagy are mentioned, there is no warning as with the English search query.

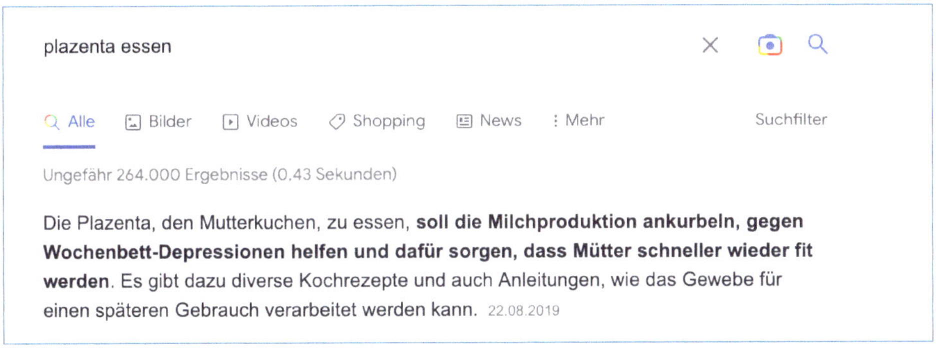

A search query on April 24, 2023 at www.google.de

"Eating the placenta is said to stimulate milk production, helps against postpartum depression and ensures that mothers become fit again more quickly. There are various recipes and instructions on how to process the tissue for later use."

Our conclusion from these examples is that search engines can be a helpful tool. However, you cannot necessarily arrive at a personal, differentiated opinion based on their algorithms. Information on the Internet is not free from the prejudices of the people who wrote the texts. The content may or may not be true.

On the one hand, "science" is currently experiencing a huge hype. People no longer rely on their own common sense, but only believe in an "expert opinion". However, with regard to the popular attitude "I love science", we think: "We love *questioning* science" - because we have to put the content we read into the appropriate context, check it for realism, critically question it and compare it with our own level of knowledge. Moreover, scientific findings are only valid for the moment and are sometimes outdated by the time they are published.

Thinking for yourself is of course exhausting - but we can't avoid it if we want to track down the truth and protect ourselves from mere "rumination".

Where are the female questions in science?

After researching the literature, we were a little surprised: The use of placenta remedies has been described for hundreds of years and documented by many sources. But there are very few clinical studies on it. Why is that?

The effort involved in a clinical study can be overcome if you want to. But who formulates the research questions? Who knows about breastfeeding problems and postpartum depression? Which (male) professor asks the female questions in science? And who funds research into women's health? Who decides on the applications for research projects?

In Germany there is still no equal distribution of male and female professors (although more women than men are now studying medicine), so who should research the topic of "postpartum"? Can "men" really imagine how a woman feels after giving birth? Sore, physically exhausted, emotionally overwhelmed, on the hormone-rollercoaster and newly confronted with the tasks of motherhood?

At the moment, the research landscape is quite "geriatric": cancer, heart disease, dementia ... Of course, good care for the elderly and sick is important, but in comparison, the attention that research pays to mothers and newborns in an absolutely vulnerable phase – which is fundamental to the health of the next generation – is negligible! Why invest so much money and time in the "end of life" when we don't even know, let alone understand, the beginning of life? How a child is born, what it experiences in the earliest phase of life, what the mother experiences and how the bond is formed – this not only has an impact on individual mother-child health, but also on the whole new society that is born and in which we will all live together.

Fortunately, there are increasingly more and more women, midwives, scientists, doctors and professors who are tackling female research issues in depth, are passionate about their topics and are working on them with superpower and female motivation. The change has begun and can no longer be stopped. In a few years, we will be able to reap the rewards ...

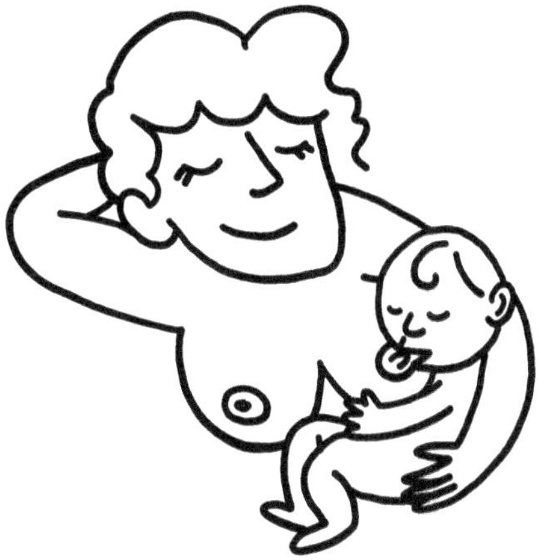

FIELD REPORT BY LINA

Unfortunately, in my training as a midwife, we never learned anything about how to use the placenta as a remedy. In fact, it was my own midwife who made me aware of this during my pregnancy. I had a complication-free pregnancy and planned to give birth to my son in a birthing center. As the pregnancy progressed, it became clear that my son would be a petite child. I had a very small belly and in fact my son was born weighing only 2,800 grams. To encourage the milk to come in, my midwife offered me to make a placenta smoothie straight after the birth. And lo and behold, less than thirty hours later I had my milk come in! My son hardly lost any weight as there was enough milk right from the start. My recovery was amazingly fast in the first few days, and I felt incredibly fit, both physically and mentally, despite the very long birth.

I was immediately enthusiastic about placentophagy and desperate to find out more. I read a lot about it in the postpartum period and also spoke to my midwife again about her experiences, the methods of administration and so on ...

After my parental leave, I went back to work. I support couples during pregnancy and in the postpartum period and give courses for first-time mothers. The placenta is a big topic at every partner evening that deals with the birth experience. Many couples have already heard that some women ingest their placenta. Nevertheless, almost everyone looks shocked at first when I tell them about placenta smoothies. However, this facial expression quickly disappears when it becomes clear why it is done and what positive effects it can have. In most of my antenatal classes, there are some couples who decide to take the placenta with them after the birth.

In the first few days postpartum, I make the women a smoothie with frozen berries, bananas, orange juice and a piece of placenta. There hasn't been one yet who hasn't liked it. One thing is always clear to see: Whether immediately after the birth or later on, milk production increases significantly. I have observed that this usually happens in the twenty-four hours after ingestion. That's why I advise every couple to take two or three pieces of placenta with them, even if the mother has perhaps not yet planned to ingest them. But if you do end up in a situation during the postpartum period where you need placenta, then it's always good to have some frozen to be on the safe side. Because sometimes the little home remedies are simply not enough to increase the amount of milk, and then a placenta smoothie is a better alternative than bottle-feeding.

But it's not just the milk let down or the increase in milk that I have had good experiences with using placenta. The smoothie also sometimes works wonders with lochial congestion, i.e. reduced postpartum bleeding.

To summarize, I can only say that the placenta can perhaps do much more than we think and is not only a faithful companion for our growing child during pregnancy, but also a valuable support for the mother in the postpartum period.

AND NOW ONCE AGAIN IN PLAIN LANGUAGE – IS THE WHOLE THING SUPPOSED TO ACHIEVE SOMETHING?

As a doctor or scientist, we cannot make a statement about placentophagy that is set in stone. This is because the scientific data is very thin on the ground. Proponents and critics can still discuss intensively the pros and cons of placenta as a remedy. But of course we can't hide the fact that we are becoming more and more enthusiastic about the topic and, after in-depth research into the literature, we believe: Yes, there certainly is something to it! Nevertheless, there is a lack of further clinical studies. In the overall view of the literature to date and the few available studies (including the limitations of these studies), it is likely that placenta as a remedy has an effect. This has also been confirmed by women in surveys from both Germany and the US.

However, we have to look at each woman individually and cannot make generalized statements. If there are women who wish to breastfeed (and want to promote milk production in a natural way) or want to regain their strength in the postpartum period, then there are various therapies and forms of support. A complex situation such as the postpartum period requires a team to meet the needs of mother and child. This includes many different professions working hand in hand, such as midwives, doulas, obstetricians, psychologists and family therapists, acupuncturists, lactation consultants, phytotherapists, osteopaths, aromatherapists, homeopaths and Phyto therapists. In addition, the individual social environment, the "personal village", is of course very important. And perhaps the placenta with its healing power is also part of this. But it doesn't have to be ...

Regardless of medical or scientific opinion, if a friend asked us confidentially and privately, we would suggest the following: "Of course, take your placenta with you for now. Because if you need it, you can always make use of its power in an emergency. Taking the placenta will almost certainly stimulate milk production. You may also subjectively experience a faster recovery and feel stronger and more balanced. This is a very valuable, endogenous remedy for the early postpartum period. And if you dry it and grind it into powder, you can use it throughout the entire breastfeeding period if you run out of milk. When the first baby year is over, put the powder in the freezer and save the contained placental hormones for the menopause ..."

To the question "How do I dose the intake?" we would have to answer: "No idea. Every placenta has an individual composition - and we can't say how much or how little you need to take. Some women take two capsules three times a day. For others, one capsule a day is enough. In the early postpartum period, it may make more sense to drink one smoothie a day. Try it out, preferably with the support of an experienced midwife. And above all: Always listen very carefully to yourself and to your body."

Midwife Cornelia Enning also differentiates the use of the personal placenta remedy on the basis of a wide range of information: What was the pregnancy like, at what time was the placenta born, is it the placenta of a boy or a girl and how many times has the mother given birth? Based on close monitoring during the pregnancy and the characteristics of the placenta that was born, she can differentiate the indications where the placenta can have the greatest effect. Some women report that they feel stressed after taking their placenta - and this could be due to the concentration of stress hormones stored in the placenta during birth.

And even if you say, despite all the hormones measured, the women only experience a placebo effect - so what? The risk of placenta ingestion is negligible, but the benefit for the child of having a happy mother is significant.

And if you're curious now, you're welcome to try it out ...

FIELD REPORT BY BERIT

My sixth and last birth in the summer of 2016, including the subsequent postpartum and breastfeeding period, seems unthinkable to me today without the supportive intake of placenta. After giving birth, I had hot flushes and sweats. Every evening, my husband gave me a smoothie with a piece of frozen placenta prepared by the midwife. After just four days, my hormone levels had regulated so that I was coping well.

In the late postpartum period, when everyday life with all its challenges had resumed, my legs often hurt due to exhaustion. Again I resorted to the placenta smoothies in the evening and already felt the following morning that the pain had subsided significantly and that I was more rested, even stronger. The smoothies made from dark berries, vanilla ice cream and a small piece of placenta were also effective when I developed breast inflammation due to changes in milk or irregularities in my daily routine. In the meantime, it has been almost six months since the birth, I have had homeopathic medicine made up and take them as needed.

However, my placenta consumption started back in 2008 after the birth of my fourth child, whom I gave birth to at home with a midwife. She let the umbilical cord pulsate out, separated the newborn from it and offered me a piece of placenta that was about the size of the nail of my little finger. I still clearly remember the taste of strawberry when I ate it. At that time, I only had it once. The postpartum period and breastfeeding went absolutely smoothly.

I took another single dose of placenta during the subsequent home birth of my daughter in May 2012. However, shortly after the birth I developed a fever due to a streptococcal infection, which was first brought under control with antibiotics in hospital. When I think back, I wonder whether the placenta would have offered a chance of recovery back then, too. I gave birth to my three older children in hospitals in 2001, 2004 and 2006, where the placenta was unfortunately discarded because I was completely unfamiliar with its benefits. And so I am both happy and grateful that it is now being taken into consideration. I myself read quite a bit about its history and value before the last birth, thanks to a friend's recommendation, and I share my experiences whenever I have the opportunity, confident that every child's placenta will return to where it belongs: in the consciousness and legacy of every family.

FOR NEW FATHERS: THE RECIPE CORNER

Anyone considering processing their own placenta at home should take into account a few requirements: it is important that neither the mother nor the child has a serious infection. It also makes sense to think about what you want to do with the placenta ahead of the birth. If you want to take it with you, it is best to take a clean, well-sealed container (don't forget to write your name on it) with you to the place of birth. The placenta can remain at room temperature for about two to four hours after the birth, then it should be placed in the refrigerator.

When the baby and placenta have just been born and the mother is perhaps exhausted and flooded with emotions, the father (or alternatively the midwife, doula, sister, mother, friend or whoever dares to take on this sometimes somewhat bloody but really special task) can take care of the placenta. This requires time, peace and quiet and a few utensils.

Preparation

The placenta must be processed in a clean kitchen. Hands should be washed before starting and it is advisable to wear gloves. It is best to use boiled stainless steel cutting tools and a cutting board that can easily be cleaned in a 90-degree dishwasher cycle. A roll of tear-resistant kitchen paper to dab the placenta dry is also necessary.

There can be something very beautiful, magical and spooky about processing the placenta in a kitchen and being in contact with this organ when you know that a new human being has just begun life through its power. Perhaps mother and child are lying in the room next door, exhausted and happy after a home birth ...

With a little reverence, a candle, a glass of wine or possibly the presence and help of a loved one, the placenta will process better. The thoughts and inner attitude towards the placenta may also have an effect on the "finished product".

And one more important note: sometimes a woman can feel a pulling sensation in her abdomen when the placenta is being processed, similar to period pain or labor pains. Therefore, a little caution is advised during pregnancy if you hold your nose close to the placenta. This is because the uterus may react when there are so many hormones in the air. Unless you want to induce birth as a self-experiment, then "sniffing the placenta" is of course allowed.

Now the mother has to decide ...

What is the best thing for the mother to do? Take her placenta raw so that the concentration of hormones is at its highest? Or process it into a food or capsule?

The decision is of course up to the woman, and it depends on which form of intake she prefers and how the dosage affects her.

We scientists are only well versed in the processing of dehydrated samples from the placenta – just as we did in the laboratory. Therefore we took the recipe for the postpartum soup from nutritionist Nathalie Stadelmann and added a piece of placenta to the soup. Theoretically, however, you can also modify any recipe for preparing meat and use the placenta instead of, for example, beef – if you like ... We look forward to hearing about your experiences!

Raw – the smoothie

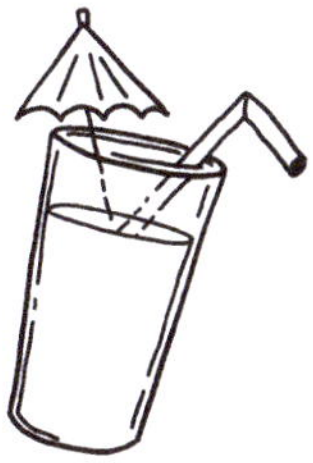

The following procedure has proven effective for taking placenta as a smoothie in the early postpartum period: Shortly after the placenta is born, about ten small pieces (about the size of a hazelnut) are cut out of the placenta and single pieces frozen in a container for ice cubes. It is simple if you use the anatomical structure of the cotyledon (see chapter *Placenta basics*), then the tissue can be easily separated out.

This means that a raw piece of placenta can be removed from the freezer and used in a fresh smoothie every day if required.

Sweet

- 1 piece of raw placenta (hazelnut sized)
- 1 handful of frozen dark berries (e.g. blueberries)
- 1/2 banana
- 200 ml mild fruit juice or tea
- 1 tsp oil (optional, for example linseed oil)

Puree the piece of placenta with the berries in a blender or chopper until you have a smooth, homogeneous puree. Then add the banana, puree well and gradually pour in juice or tea until the desired drinking liquid is achieved.

Savory

- 1 piece of raw placenta (hazelnut sized))
- 200 ml tomato juice or other vegetable juice
- 1 teaspoon olive oil
- Cucumber or celery as decoration

Puree the piece of placenta in a blender with 3 to 4 tablespoons of juice until you have a smooth, homogeneous puree. Then slowly pour in the rest of the juice, add the oil and continue to blend until the desired consistency is achieved. Garnish with sliced cucumber or celery.

Postpartum soup

- 200 g carrots
- 100 g parsnips
- 200 g fennel
- 20 g ginger
- 1 piece of placenta (hazelnut sized))
- 1 organic broiler (chicken for soup)
- 1 teaspoon caraway seeds
- 1 teaspoon fennel seeds
- 1 sprig of rosemary
- 1 teaspoon Angelica sinensis root, chopped
- Juice of 1 organic lemon
- Sea salt
- Yeast flakes

Wash and peel or clean the vegetables. Cut into large pieces. Peel and finely slice the ginger. Wash the chicken under cold running water and place it in a pan with the piece of placenta, vegetables, ginger, caraway seeds, fennel seeds, rosemary sprig and angelica root. Pour in enough cold water to cover everything.

Bring the soup to the boil. Then simmer over a low heat for at least 1 1/2 hours. Remove the meat, vegetables and spices from the stock with a slotted spoon. Remove the meat from the bones, cut into bite-sized pieces and return to the stock. Also cut the piece of placenta into very small pieces. Season each portion with a little lemon juice, sea salt and yeast flakes before serving.

You can add boiled pasta, semolina dumplings, pancake strips, barley pearl or even a whisked egg or egg dip to the soup.

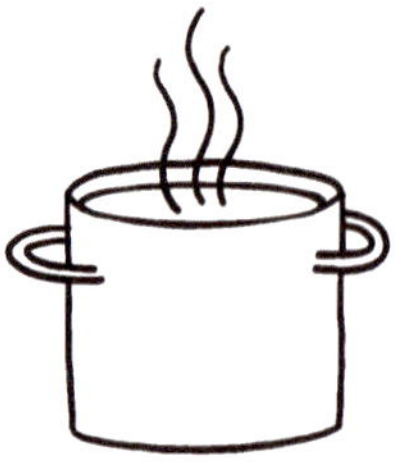

Production of placenta powder

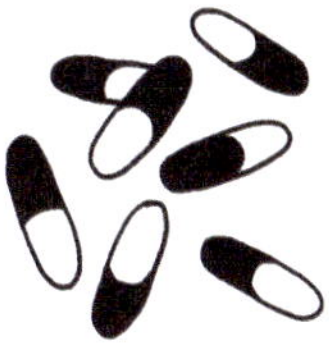

If you want to dehydrate and pulverize the placenta, there are two options: steamed/dehydrated or dehydrated only.

Steamed

Not all sources of Chinese medicine mention that the placenta should be steamed before drying. But it is of course a good method to kill microorganisms. It just smells intensely in the kitchen - that's why we always worked under the extractor hood in the laboratory.

You need:

- Steamer pot
- approx. 3 to 4 cm ginger
- 1/2 lime, quartered
- Aluminum foil

Bring the water, ginger and lime to the boil. Place the placenta in the top of the steamer. Do not place the organ directly on the stainless steel, otherwise it may bake: Form a basket or nest from aluminum foil and place the raw placenta on top.

It is then steamed - until the internal temperature in the center of the placenta exceeds 70 degrees Celsius and no more blood is visible when you press on the placenta with a fork. Allow the piece to cool thoroughly and then cut it into thin slices of around 0.5 to 1.0 centimeter for drying in a dehydrator or oven.

Dehydrated

The placenta strips are dehydrated at 55 degrees Celsius for eight hours. You can either use a dehydrator or the oven (then put a wooden spoon in the door so that the moisture can escape).

First, line the inserts of the dehydrator or the baking tray with baking paper. The placenta is either cut into 0.5 to 1.0 cm thin strips while still raw or already steamed. Place these stripes of tissue on the baking paper with a little space between them. Then leave them to dry.

After eight hours, carry out the "snap test": The tissue should be easy to break when it is completely dry. If it is still somewhat pliable, continue the dehydration for a further two hours.

The dehydrated strips can then be ground into powder in a food processor. Store this in a dark glass jar in a place protected from light. If you have empty capsules from the pharmacy, it is best to fill all the capsules at once with the powder (capsules of 500 milligrams are often used) so that you don't keep contaminating the powder with your hands through repeated fillings.

Our tests have shown that storing the placenta powder for six months in a dry, dark place poses no risk of microbial growth. In plain language: the powder does not spoil after six months. The capsules can also be frozen if they are not needed for the time being.

Preparation of a placenta tincture

Perhaps there are also women who do not like it quite so "organic" and prefer to take their placenta in an abstract form. In this case, you can have homeopathic medicine made from your own placenta in various potencies in specialized German pharmacies. Another option is the homeopathic tincture.

The procedure for preparing a mother tincture is described in detail in the European Homeopathic Pharmacopoeia. It involves dynamizing and diluting the original substance. According to the pharmacist Samuel Hahnemann, a substance can be changed by rubbing and shaking it so that it unfolds "the revelation of the specific medicinal powers hidden in their essence". This is why he developed the process of dynamization. The standardized dilution merely served to avoid the side effects of toxic starting materials.

Making a placenta tincture is not very complicated. The steps are briefly and concisely summarized here. The preparation of the potentization steps according to Korsakow is a traditional method and cannot be found in the Homeopathic Pharmacopoeia.

The tinctures produced and the raw materials required should be kept away from children. Caution: Tinctures have a high alcohol content and should therefore only be taken by children and recovered alcoholics in consultation with a doctor or pharmacist. You should only add the tincture drop by drop to a glass of water if you want to take it.

If you want to make your own placenta tincture, you don't need much:

- a clean kitchen, washed hands, knife, chopping board and tweezers (preferably scalded once with boiling water and thus as germ-free as possible)
- a cleaned, dark glass jar with a screw cap
- a fine tea strainer
- a clean glass with a spout
- one dark glass bottle (15 ml)
- 85% glycerol (can be ordered from pharmacies)
- high-proof alcohol, for example 30% ethanol (can be ordered from pharmacies)
- 1 thumbnail-sized piece of fresh placenta
- Label

The first step is to prepare a mother tincture. A mother tincture should contain as much information as possible from the original substance. This is why raw placenta is used, the fresher the better. This starting substance is prepared in a ratio of 1:9 in 85% glycerol. A piece of placenta about the size of a thumbnail is cut into very small pieces on a chopping board with a knife and then filled into the jar with a screw cap using tweezers. This small amount of placenta corresponds to one part of the starting substance.

Now add 9 parts of the glycerol. It is important to ensure that the tissue is completely covered, otherwise it may spoil. The bottle is only filled up to ✥ full, no more. Now store this mixture in a dark place for at least five days. It is then filtered: The glycerol extract is poured through a fine tea strainer into a clean glass with a spout. The mother tincture is ready! This corresponds to the 1st decimal dilution (= D1).

The 2nd decimal dilution D2 is prepared from one part mother tincture (D1) and nine parts ethanol (30 %): Take the small brown glass bottle and fill it with about 1 to 2 milliliters of the mother tincture. Ethanol is then added in a ratio of 1:9. The brown glass bottle now contains a placenta tincture in the decimal dilution D2.

Single glass method according to Korsakow

Hahnemann used a new bottle for each dilution step. However, the more potency levels you want to produce, the more costly and uneconomical it is to purchase many glass bottles. Simeon Korsakov, who treated many patients with homeopathy during a cholera epidemic between 1841 and 1844, therefore revised Hahnemann's method and simplified it.

According to Korsakow, dynamization and dilution are carried out in one and the same bottle, filled up to 3/4 full. This is based on the adhesive force that exists between the vessel wall and the medicinal liquid and ensures that a drop of liquid always remains in the glass. In addition to dilution, dynamization is also important: This involves shaking the bottle vigorously at least ten times (preferably with strong strikes on a pillow or a towel folded several times). Dynamization is started with the bottle containing the placenta tincture D2:

- Dynamize (several strong strikes of the bottle on a cushion)
- Now empty the contents of the bottle with a strong-arm stroke (this ensures that only one drop remains inside the bottle due to adhesion).
- This is followed by the 1:100 dilution (centimal dilution): 99 drops of alcohol are added to the one remaining drop in the now "empty" bottle (if you are an exact person, count the drops - then the dilution is exact. Otherwise you can simply refill the bottle up to ✥ full with alcohol).
- Dynamize again: Shake or bump the bottle vigorously ten times (at this point the bottle contains the placenta tincture C1)
- Empty the contents of the bottle again with a vigorous arm movement
- Fill up with 99 drops of alcohol (dilution 1:200 - i.e. C2)
- Repeat shaking and diluting until the result is C3

The processes of dynamization and dilution can now be continued as desired up to the desired potency.

Finally, put a label on the jar: Write down the date of manufacture and the dilution of the placenta tincture. Done!

APPENDIX

From: Johnson, S. K., Pastuschek, J., Benyshek, D. C., Heimann, Y., Möller, A., Rödel, J., White, J., Zöllkau, J., Groten, T. (2022): "Impact of tissue processing on microbiological colonization in the context of placentophagy". In: Sci Rep 12 (1): 5307: Microorganisms on raw, steamed, raw/dheydrated and steamed/dehydrated placenta preparations (n=24). This study investigates the maternal colonization with B Streptococci (GBS).

<table>
<tr><th></th><th>Birth mode</th><th>Antibiotic treatment</th><th>raw</th></tr>
<tr><td rowspan="3">GBS-positive according to maternity record</td><td rowspan="2">Vaginal delivery</td><td>no</td><td>Kocuria kristinae, Corynebacterium spp., Coagulase-negative Staphylococci, Streptococcus anginosus, Staphylococcus epidermidis, Cryptococcus sedentarius, Pseudomonas aeruginosa</td></tr>
<tr><td>Yes</td><td>Achromobacter xylosoxidans*</td></tr>
<tr><td>C-Section</td><td>no</td><td>Gardnarella vaginalis</td></tr>
<tr><td rowspan="2">Unscreened for GBS</td><td>Vaginal delivery</td><td>no</td><td>Staphylococcus haemolyticus, Staphylococcus epidermidis, Cutibacterium acnes</td></tr>
<tr><td>C-Section</td><td>no</td><td>Staphylococcus lugdunensis, Staphylococcus epidermidis</td></tr>
</table>

- means no growth after 48 hours

* *Achromobacter xylosoxidans*: This bacterium was a contaminant, contamination occurred during sample processing. Achromobacter xylosoxidans was detected in the tap water and also in the surface disinfectant.

steamed	**raw/dehydrated**	**steamed/ dehydrated**
Staphylococcus warneri	*Staphylococcus epidermidis*	-
Paenibacillus pabuli, Staphylococcus epidermidis, *Achromobacter xylosoxidans**	*Staphylococcus epidermidis, Micrococcus luteus*	-
Micrococcus luteus	*Propionibacterium acnes*	-
Staphylococcus epidermidis, Cutibacterium acnes	*Corynebacterium tuberculo-stearicum, Staphylococcus epidermidis*	*Bacillus subtilis*
Bacilllus subtilis, Staphylococcus pasteuri, Staphylococcus epider-midis, Paenibacillus lautus	*Cutibacterium acnes*	*Paenibacillus provencensis*

Johnson S.K., Groten, T., Pastuschek, J., Rödel J., Sammer, U., Markert, U.R. (2018): "Human placentophagy: Effects of dehydration and steaming on hormones, metals and bacteria in placental tissue". In: Placenta 67: 8-14. This table shows microorganisms isolated from samples of raw, raw dehydrated and steamed dehydrated placental tissue.

Retained samples were analyzed after 6 month (+/- 8 weeks)

Sample Number	Swab fetal side	Swab maternal side	Raw	Steamed
P2	*Lactobacillaceae, Staphylococcus haemolyticus*	*Lactobacillaceae, Staphylcoccus haemolyticus*	*'Lactobacillaceae, Corynebacterium spp, Burkholderia gladioli*	*Staphylococcus haemolyticus, Corynebacterium spp*
P3	Coagulase-negative Staphylococci, Streptococcus anginosus	Coagulase-negative Staphylococci, Gardnerella vaginalis	*Escherichia coli, Gardnerella vaginalis*	-
P4	*Lactobacillaceae, Coagulase-negative Staphylococci, Streptococcus anginosus, Candida albicans, Micrococcaceae, Bifidobacterium ssp., Prevotella spp.*	*Lactobacillaceae, Staphylococcus epidermidis, Bifidobacterium ssp.*	*Lactobacillaceae, Staphylococcus epidermidis, Streptococcus anginosus*	*Enterococcus faecalis, Achromomobacter xylosoxidans**
P5	Coagulase-negative Staphylococci, Streptococcus anginosus, Achromomobacter xylosoxidans*, Corynebacterium spp., Gardnerella vaginalis, Peptococcaceae	Coagulase-negative Staphylococci, Streptococcus anginosus, Corynebacterium spp., Haemophilus parainfluenzae, Bacteroides thetaiotaomicron, Peptostreptococcus	*Lactobacillaceae, Streptococcus anginosus, Achromomobacter xylosoxidans*, Bacteroides spp., Capnocytophaga spp., Peptostreptococcus*	*Achromomobacter xylosoxidans**
P6	*Lactobacillaceae, Staphylococcus epidermidis, Candida albicans*	*Lactobacillaceae, Staphylococcus epidermidis, Candida albicans*	*Lactobacillaceae, Candida albicans, Achromomobacter xylosoxidans**	*Achromomobacter xylosoxidans**
P7	Coagulase-negative Staphylococci, Corynebacterium spp.	Coagulase-negative Staphylococci	*Corynebacterium spp.*	-
P8	*Enterococcus faecalis, Candida albicans*	*Lactobacillaceae, Coagulase-negative Staphylococci, Candida albicans*	Coagulase-negative Staphylococci	-
P9	-	-	-	-
Number of different species	**14**	**12**	**13**	**4**

spp. Means species pluralis, several species of a genus

- = no growth after 48 hours

* means contamination (this contaminant was found in the tap water and disinfectant of the lab)

Raw/dehydrated	Steamed/dehydrated	Raw/dehydrated retained sample (4° Celsius)	Raw/dehydrated retained sample (room temperature)	Steamed/dehydrated retained sample (4° Celsius)	Steamed/dehydrated retained sample (room temperature)
-	*Staphylococcus haemolyticus, Corynebacterium spp*	-	-	-	-
'*Pantoea agglomerans*	-	-	-	-	-
'*Lactobacillaceae, Coagulase-negative Staphylococci, Streptococcus anginosus, Streptococcus mitis/ oralis*	-	*Lactobacillaceae, Coagulase-negative Staphylococci, Proprionibacteria*	-	*Bacillus spp.*	-
-	-	-	-	*Paenibacillus macerans*	*Paenibacillus macerans*
-	-	*Roseomonas mucosa*	*Paenibacillus macerans*	-	*Paenibacillus macerans*
Coagulase-negative Staphylococci	-	Coagulase-negative Staphylococci	-	-	-
-	-	-	Coagulase-negative Staphylococci	-	-
-	-	-	-	-	-
5	**2**	**4**	**2**	**2**	**1**

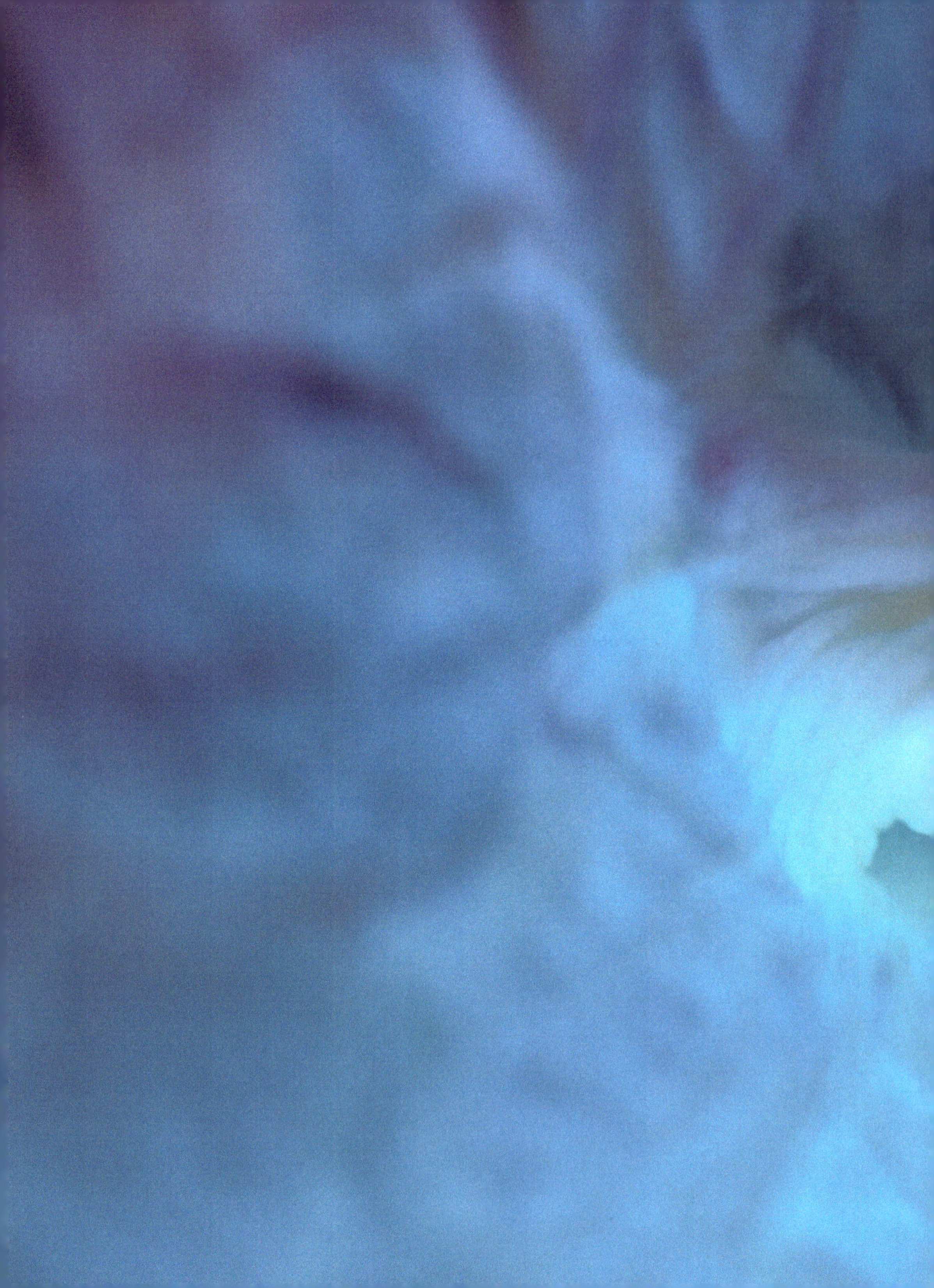

REFERENCES

Introduction to our placenta universe

Enning, C. (2003): *Heilmittel aus Plazenta. Medizinisches und Ethnomedizinisches.* Norderstedt: Books on Demand.

Farr, A. et al (2018): "Human placentophagy: a review". In: *Am J Obstet Gynecol* 218 (4): 401-411.

Münz, A. (2020): *Placentophagie. Erfahrungen von Andwenderinnen und Entwicklung eines Informationsblattes.* Bachelor thesis, Heidenheim (https://geburtshausansbach.de/ wpcontent/uploads/Bachelorarbeit_Plazentophagie.pdf, last accessed on 27.09.2021).

Shizhen, L. and Unschuld, P.U. (editor and translator) (2021): *Ben Cao Gang Mu. Volume IX: Fowls, Domestic and Wild Animals, Human Substances.* Berkeley, Los Angeles: University of California Press.

The placenta: miracle organ and all-rounder

Aagaard, K. et al. (2014): "The placenta harbors a unique microbiome". In: *Sci Transl Med:* 21; 6 (237): 237ra65.

Bushman, F.D. (2019): "De-Discovery of the Placenta Microbiome". In: *Am J Obstet Gynecol* 220 (3): 213–214.

Chrousos, G.P. et al. (1998): "Interactions between the hypothalamicpituitaryadrenal axis and the female reproductive system: clinical implications". In: *Ann Intern Med* 129 (3): 229–240.

Cohain, J.S. (2022): "Novel third stage protocol https://www.youtube.com/watch?v=AAJPW4p6rzU reduces postpartum hemorrhage at vaginal birth". In: *Eur J Obstet Gynecol Reprod Biol* Volume 278: 29–32.

Dudenhausen, J.W. (2011): *Praktische Geburtshilfe mit geburtshilflichen Operationen.* 21st expanded edition, Berlin: Walter de Gruyter & Co.

Evain-Brion, D. and Malassine, A. (2003): "Human placenta as an endocrine organ". In: *Growth Hormone and IGF Research* 13 Suppl. A: 34–37.

Huppertz, B. and Schleußner, E. (eds.) (2018): *Die Plazenta. Grundlagen und klinische Bedeutung.* Heidelberg: Springer Verlag.

NIH Human Microbiome Project (https://hmpdacc.org/, last accessed on 03.05.2023).

Norman, A.W. and Litwack, G. (1997): "Hormones". In: *Academic Press*: 387–411.

Reis, F.M. and Petraglia, F. (2001): "The placenta as a neuroendocrine organ". In: *Frontiers of Hormone Research* 27: 216–228.

Schad, W. (ed.) (2008): *Die verlorene Hälfte des Menschen. Die Plazenta vor und nach der Geburt in Medizin, Ethnologie und Anthroposophie.* 2nd improved edition, Stuttgart: Verlag Freies Geistesleben.

Schulkin, J. and Power, M.L. (2012): *The Evolution of the Human Placenta.* Baltimore: Johns Hopkins University Press.

Tchuitcheu, J.K. (2010): *Die Versorgung der menschlichen Nachgeburt als Spiegel ihres ethno-medizinischen Stellenwertes weltweit.* Dissertation, Berlin: Salumed Verlag (https://www.salumedverlag.de/files/bilder/Downloaddateien/Final_Dissertation.pdf, last accessed on 14.02.2023).

Vidal, A. and Peric, A. (2022): "The important role of the microbiome in the female genital tract and its impact on fertility". In: *J Reproductive Med Endocri- nol* 19 (2): 78–84.

The ritual use of the placenta

Ade-Rademacher, D. et al. (1997): *Wo weder Sonne noch Mond hinscheint. Archäologische Nachweise von Nachgeburtsbestattungen in der frühen Neuzeit.* Stuttgart (= Archäologische Informationen aus Baden Württemberg, Heft 36, published by Landesamt für Denkmalpflege im Regierungspräsidium Stuttgart).

Bächtold-Stäubli, H. (1934/1935/1986): *Handwörterbuch des deutschen Aberglaubens.* Berlin: Walter de Gruyter & Co.

Kuntner, L. (2004): "Zum Umgang mit der Nachgeburt. Plazentabestattung im Kulturverlgeich". In: *Curare* 27 (3): 279–293.

Moser, D.A. (2019): *Wurzel des Lebens. Die menschliche Plazenta vor und nach der Geburt.* Wien: Morawa Lesezirkel.

Schad, W. (ed.) (2008): *Die verlorene Hälfte des Menschen. Die Plazenta vor und nach der Geburt in Medizin, Ethnologie und Anthroposophie.* 2nd improved edition, Stuttgart: Verlag Freies Geistesleben.

Shizhen, L. and Unschuld, P. U. (editor and translator) (2021): *Ben Cao Gang Mu. Volume IX: Fowls, Domestic and Wild Animals, Human Substances.* Berkeley, Los Angeles: University of California Press.

Tchuitcheu, J. K. (2010): *Die Versorgung der menschlichen Nachgeburt als Spiegel ihres ethno-medizinischen Stellenwertes weltweit.* Dissertation, Berlin: Salumed Verlag (https://www.salumedverlag.de/files/bilder/Downloaddateien/Final_Dissertation.pdf, last accessed on 14.02.2023).

History and curiosities

Chochlow, A. W. (1921): "Die Plazenta als Heilmittel in der Volksmedizin". In: *Zentralblatt für Gynäkologie* 27: 1497–1501.

Dettling, A. (1911): "Arzneibuch Landammans Michael Schorno von Schwyz (died 1671)". In: *Schweizer Archiv für Volkskunde* 15: 89–94, 177–184.

Enning, C. (2003): *Heilmittel aus Plazenta. Medizinisches und Ethnomedizinisches* Norderstedt: Books on Demand.

Gesner, J. A. M. and Mauchart, B. D. (1741): *Pharmacopoea Wirtenbergica: In Duas Partes Divisa, Quarum prior, Materiam Medicam, Historico-Physico-Medice Descriptam, Posterior, Composita Et Praeparata, Modum Praeparandi Et Encheireses, Exhibet. Iussu Serenissimi Domini Ducis Adornata, Et Pharmacopoeis Wirtenbergicis In Normam Praescripta.* Stuttgart: Verlag Erhard.

Jütte, R. (2009): "Organpräparate in der Geschichte der Schulmedizin, Homöopathie und Anthroposophischen Medizin". In: *Der Merkurstab* 62 (1): 49–60.

Les Laboratoires Homoeopathiques de France (ed.) (1949): *Documentations Homoeopathiques XVII,* Paris.

Möslein, P. (1949): *Die Behandlung der secundären Amenorrhoe mit Frischdrüseneinreibungen (Ovar, Placenta).* Dissertation, Friedrich Schiller University Jena.

Ober, W. B. (1979): "Notes on placentophagy". In: *Bull N Y Acad Med* 55 (6): 591–599.

Steiner, R. and Wegman, I. (1991): *Grundlegendes für eine Erweiterung der Heilkunst nach geisteswissenschaftlichen Erkenntnissen.* 7th edition, Dornach: Rudolf Steiner Verlag.

Placenta as a remedy

Bensky, D. et al. (1986): Chinese herbal Medicine: *Materia medica.* Seattle: Eastland Press.

Biggs, K. and Gwillim, M. (2000): *Placenta humanum (Welsh)* (https://welshschoolof homeopathy.org.uk/provings/Placenta.pdf, last accessed 13.03.2023).

Hahnemann, S. (2005): *Organon der Heilkunst. Das Standardwerk der Homöopathie.* 6th edition, Wiesbaden: Marix Verlag.

Homöopathisches Arzneibuch (2022): Stuttgart: Deutscher Apotheker Verlag.

Jütte, R. (2009): "Organpräparate in der Geschichte der Schulmedizin, Homöopathie und Anthroposophischen Medizin". In: *Der Merkurstab* 62 (1): 49-60.

Kunkel, M. and Wiesenauer, M. (2013): "Plazenta-Nosoden: eine Dokumentation". In: *Midwifery Forum* 14: 713-716.

Nagase, M. et al. (2020): "Improvement of Aspects of Subjective Sleep Quality of Healthy Volunteers by Ingestion of Porcine Placental Extract: A Randomized Cross Over Pilot Study". In: *Front. Nutr* 7: 550287.

Pan, S. et al. (2017): "Placental Therapy: An insight to their biological and therapeutic properties". In: *J Med Therap* 1: 1-6.

Schad, W. (ed.) (2008): *Die verlorene Hälfte des Menschen. Die Plazenta vor und nach der Geburt in Medizin, Ethnologie und Anthroposophie.* 2nd improved edition, Stuttgart: Verlag Freies Geistesleben.

Schad, W. (2016): unpublished correspondence in the possession of the author Sophia Johnson.

Shizhen, L. and Unschuld, P. U. (editor and translator) (2021): *Ben Cao Gang Mu. Volume IX: Fowls, Domestic and Wild Animals, Human Substances.* Berkeley, Los Angeles: University of California Press.

Soldner, G. (2004): "Zur Therapie mit potenzierten embryonalen Organpräparaten: Amnion, Funiculus umbilicalis, Placenta". In: *Merkurstab* 57 (5): 373-374.

Steiner, R. and Wegman, I. (1991): *Grundlegendes für eine Erweiterung der Heilkunst nach geisteswissenschaftlichen Erkenntnissen.* 7th edition, Dornach: Rudolf Steiner Verlag.

Stux, G. (2020): *Akupunktur – Heilen mit Energiemedizin. Akupunkur-Publikationen aus 10 Jahren Naturheilkunde Journal.* Bamberg: MLVerlag.

Wittwer, H. (2019): *Muttermittel in der täglichen Praxis.* Kilchberg: Timia Verlag.

Zerm, C. (2023): Interview with the author Sophia Johnson on 21.01.2023, unpublished recording in the author's possession.

Placentophagy

Benyshek, D. C. (2019): Conversation with the author Sophia Johnson after the lecture "Human maternal placentophagy: evolutionary roots, cross-cultural occurrence, and an emerging postindustrial health trend" on March 14, 2019, unpublished notes in possession of the author.

Benyshek, D. C. et al. (2018): "Placentophagy among women planning community births in the United States: Frequency, rationale, and associated neonatal outcomes". In: *Birth* 45 (4): 459–468.

Blank, M. S. and Friesen, H. G. (1980): "Effects of placentophagy on serum prolactin and progesterone concentrations in rats after parturition or superovulation". In: *J Reprod Fertil* 60: 273–278.

Botelle, R. and Willott, C. (2020): "Birth, attitudes and placentophagy: a thematic discourse analysis of discussions on UK parenting forums". In: *BMC Pregnancy and Childbirth* 20: 134.

Bush, P. G. et al. (2000): "A quantitative study on the effects of maternal smoking on placental morphology and cadmium concentration". In: *Placenta* 21 (2–3): 247–256.

Gélis, J. (1989): *Die Geburt. Volksglaube, Rituale und Praktiken von 1500–1900.* München: Diederichs.

Johnson S. K., Groten, T., Pastuschek, J., Rödel, J., Sammer, U., Markert, U. R. (2018): "Human placentophagy: Effects of dehydration and steaming on hormones, metals and bacteria in placental tissue". In: *Placenta* 67: 8–14.

Kristal, M. B. (1980): "Placentophagia: a biobehavioral enigma (or De gustibus non disputandum est)". In: *Neurosci Biobehav Rev* 4 (2): 141–150.

Kristal, M. B. et al. (2012): "Placentophagia in humans and nonhuman mammals: causes and consequences". In: *Ecol Food Nutr* 51 (3): 177–197.

Mozart Letters and Documents – Online Edition, published by the International Mozarteum Foundation, Salzburg (https://dme.mozarteum.at/briefedokumente, last accessed on 14.04.2023).

Ober, W. B. (1968): "A Modest Proposal for Preventing Choriocarcinoma among Innocent Mothers". In: *Obstet Gynecol* 31 (6): 866–869.

Schmidt, C. R. (1976): *Verhalten einer Zoogruppe von Halsband-Pekaris (Tayassu tajacu).* Zurich: Juris Druck & Verlag.

Selander, J. et al. (2013): "Human Maternal Placentophagy: A Survey of self-reported Motivations and Experiences Associated with Placenta Consumption". In: *Ecol Food Nutr* 52 (2): 93–115.

Sjilds, K. (1972): "1971 Birth". In: *Rolling Stone.*

Stoeverock, M. (2021): *Female Choice. Vom Anfang und Ende der männlichen Zivilisation.* Stuttgart: KlettCotta.

Tchuitcheu, J. K. (2010): *Die Versorgung der menschlichen Nachgeburt als Spiegel ihres ethno-medizinischen Stellenwertes weltweit.* Dissertation, Berlin: Salumed Verlag (https://www.salumedverlag.de/files/bilder/Downloaddateien/Final_Dissertation.pdf, last accessed on 14.02.2023).

Young, S. M. and Benyshek D. C. (2010): "In search of human placentophagy: a cross cultural survey of human placenta consumption, disposal practices, and cultural beliefs". In: *Ecol Food Nutr* 49 (6): 467–484.

Young, S. M. and Benyshek, D. C. (2012): "The Conspicuous Absence of Placenta Consumption in Human Postpartum Females: The Fire Hypothesis". In: *Ecol Food Nutr* 51 (3): 198–217.

Drug or food?

Danz, S. (2008): "Wem gehört die Nabelschnur?" In: *MedR* 26 (10): 602–607.

Donley, G. (2019): "Regulation of Encapsulated Placenta". In: *Tennessee Law Review* 86: 225–287.

The placenta as a research object

Benyshek, D. C. et al. (2018): "Placentophagy among women planning community births in the United States: Frequency, rationale, and associated neonatal outcomes". In: *Birth* 45 (4): 459–468.

Bové, H. et al. (2019): "Ambient black carbon particles reach the fetal side of human placenta". In: *Nat Commun* 10 (1): 3866.

Buser, G. L. et al. (2017): "LateOnset Infant Group B Streptococcus Infection Associa ted with Maternal Consumption of Capsules Containing Dehydrated Placenta – Oregon, 2016". In: *Morbidity and Mortality Weekly Report (MMWR)* 66 (25): 677-678.

Chang, S. et al. (2017): "Nutritional composition and heavy metal content of the human placenta". In: *Placenta* 60: 100–102.

Chrousos, G. P. et al. (1998): "Interactions between the hypothalamicpituitaryadrenal axis and the female reproductive system: clinical implications". In: *Ann Intern Med* 129 (3): 229–240.

Dalton, K. and Holton, W. (2001): *Depression after Childbirth*. 4th revised edition, Oxford: Oxford University Press.

Deutsche Gesellschaft für Ernährung e. V.: *Referenzwert Eisen* (https://www.dge.de/wissenschaft/referenzwerte/eisen/, last accessed on 11.07.2023).

Grafmüller, S. et al. (2013): "Determination of the transport rate of xenobiotics and nanomaterials across the placenta using the ex vivo human placental perfusion model". In: *J Vis Exp* (76): 50401.

Hübner-Liebermann, B. et al. (2012): "Recognizing and treating peripartum depres sion". In: *Dtsch Arztebl Int* 109 (24): 419–424.

Johnson S. K., Groten, T., Pastuschek, J., Rödel, J., Sammer, U., Markert, U. R. (2018): "Human placentophagy: Effects of dehydration and steaming on hormones, metals and bacteria in placental tissue". In: *Placenta* 67: 8–14.

Johnson, S. K. (2018): *Aspects of placentophagy: Original data and literature review.* Dissertation, Friedrich Schiller University Jena.

Johnson, S. K., Pastuschek, J., Benyshek, D. C., Heimann, Y., Möller, A., Rödel, J., White, J., Zöllkau, J., Groten, T. (2022): "Impact of tissue processing on microbiological colonization in the context of placentophagy". In: *Sci Rep* 12 (1): 5307 (https://www.nature.com/articles/s41598-022-09243-4, last accessed on 21.05.2023).

Johnson, S. K., Pastuschek, J., Heimann Y. (2022): "Placenta tissue processing protocol – in the context of placentophagy" (https://protocolexchange.research-square.com/article/pex-1888/v1, last accessed on 21.05.2023).

Jureidini, J. and McHenry, L. B. (2022): "The illusion of evidence based medicine". In: *BMJ 376: o702.*

Kanes, S. et al (2017): "Brexanolone (SAGE547 injection) in postpartum depression: a randomized controlled trial". In: *Lancet* 390 (10093): 480–489.

Madrid, L. et al. (2017): "Infant Group B Streptococcal Disease Incidence and Serotypes Worldwide: Systematic Review and Metaanalyses". In: *Clin Infect Dis.* 6; 65 (suppl_2): 160–172.

Mathiesen, L. et al (2021): "Fetal exposure to environmental chemicals; insights from placental perfusion studies". In: *Placenta* 106: 58–66.

Nelson, J. L. (2003): "Microchimerism in human health and disease". In: *Autoimmunity* 36 (1): 5–9.

Phuapradit, W. et al. (2000): "Nutrients and hormones in heatdried human placenta". In: *J Med Assoc Thai* 83 (6): 690–694.

Ragusa, A. et al (2021): "Plasticenta: First evidence of microplastics in human placen ta". In: *Environ Int.* 146: 106274.

Russell, N. J. et al. (2017): "Maternal Colonization with Group B Streptococcus and Sero-type Distribution Worldwide: Systematic Review and Metaanalyses". In: *Clin Infect Dis* 65: 100–111.

Sackett, D. L. et al. (1996): "Evidence based medicine: what it is and what it isn't". In: *BMJ* 312 (7023): 71–72.

Schneider, H. et al (2021): "Ex vivo dual perfusion of an isolated cotyledon of human placenta: History and future challenges". In: *Placenta* 107: 8–12.

Shizhen, L. and Unschuld, P. U. (editor and translator) (2021): *Ben Cao Gang Mu. Volume IX: Fowls, Domestic and Wild Animals, Human Substances.* Berkeley, Los Angeles: University of California Press.

Street, M. E. et al. (2020): "EndocrineDisrupting Chemicals in Human Fetal Growth". In: *Int J Mol Sci* 20; 21 (4): 1430.

Consumer advice center Hamburg (2023): "Harmful substances in food. Germs in meat – what to do?" (https://www.vzhh.de/themen/lebensmittelernaehrung/schad stoffelebensmitteln/keimeimfleischwastun, last accessed on 19.04.2023).

Commission Regulation (EC) No 2073/2005 of November 15, 2005 on microbiological criteria for foodstuffs, published in: *Official Journal of the European Union* L 338, 22.12.2005: 1-26.

Commission Regulation (EC) No. 1881/2006 of December 19, 2006 in the consolidated version of 01.09.2014 setting maximum levels for certain contaminants in foodstuffs, published in: *Official Journal of the European Union* L 364, 20.12.2006, 5-24.

Young, S. M. et al. (2016): "Human placenta processed for encapsulation contains modest concentrations of 14 trace minerals and elements". In: *Nutr Res* 36 (8): 872-878.

The state of research on placentophagia

(The sources listed here are those from the tabular overview on pages 141-143 that have not already been cited elsewhere).

Gryder, L. K. et al. (2017): "Effects of Human Maternal Placentophagy on Maternal Postpartum Iron Status: A Randomized, Double-Blind, Placebo-Controlled Pilot Study". In: *J Midwifery Womens Health* 62: 68-79.

Hammett, F. S. (1918): "The effect of the maternal ingestion of desiccated placenta upon the rate of growth of breastfed infants". In: *J Biol Chem* 36: 569-573.

Hammett, F. S. and McNeile, L. G. (1917): "Concerning the Effect of Ingested Placenta on the Growth-Promoting Properties of Human Milk". In: *Science* 46 (1188): 345-346.

Kristal, M. B. (1991): "Enhancement of opioid-mediated analgesia: A solution to the enigma of placentophagia". In: *Neuroscience and Biobehavioral Reviews* 15 (3): 425-435.

Interview with Udo Markert (2017): "Plazenta im Backofen". In: *DER SPIEGEL* 2: 104 (https://magazin.spiegel.de/EpubDelivery/spiegel/pdf/148899557, last accessed on 17.02.2023).

Soykova-Pachnerova, E. et al. (1954): "Placenta as a Lactagogon". In: *Gynaecologia* 138: 617-627.

Whittington, J. R. et al. (2020): "Alternative Birth Plans and Unintended Maternal and Neonatal Consequences: A Review of the Literature". In: *Obstet Gynecol Surv* Dec; 75 (12): 766-778.

Young, S. M. et al. (2016): "Presence and concentration of 17 hormones in human placenta processed for encapsulation and consumption". In: *Placenta* 43: 86-89.

Young, S. M. et al. (2018): "Effects of placentophagy on maternal salivary hormones: A pilot trial, part 1". In: *Women Birth* 31: 245-257.

Young, S. M. et al. (2018): "Placentophagy's effects on mood, bonding, and fatigue: A pilot trial, part 2". In: *Women Birth* 31: 258-271.

And now once again in plain language – is the whole thing supposed to achieve something?

Enning, C. (2003): *Remedies from placenta. Medical and ethnomedical aspects.* Norderstedt: Books on Demand.

Münz, A. (2020): Plazentophagie – *Erfahrungen von Anwenderinnen und Entwicklung eines Informationsblattes.* Bachelor thesis, Heidenheim (https://geburtshausansbach.de/wpcontent/uploads/Bachelorarbeit_Plazentophagie.pdf, last accessed on 27.09.2021).

Selander, J. et al. (2013): "Human maternal placentophagy: A survey of self-reported motivations and experiences associated with placenta consumption". In: *Ecology of Food and Nutrition* 52 (2): 93-115.

For new fathers: the recipe corner

Homöopathisches Arzneibuch (2022): Stuttgart: Deutscher Apotheker Verlag.

"Korsakow-Methode". In: Homöopedia. *Information zur Homöopathie* (https://www.homöopedia.eu/index.php/Artikel:KorsakowMethode, last accessed on 14.05.2023).

Stadelmann, N. (2021): *Ernährung in Schwangerschaft & Stillzeit.* Wiggensbach: Stadelmann Verlag.

Picture credits and sources, unless otherwise stated:

Photo Credits:

Trevor Johnson, photographer (Page 42–43, 86, 90–91, 114–115, www.trevorjohnson.de

Manuel Nagel, photographer (Page 8,18, 48–49, 58, 94,172–173 www.manuelnagel.de

Anisá Namdar, Art Director www.nisnamdarstudio.com

You can find a selection of high-quality prints at www.placentaprints.com

Illustrations

www.sandruschka.de

Further sources

P. 21/23: Prof. Dr. Wolfgang Schad "Die verlorene Hälfte des Menschen" ©: 2005 Verlag Freies Geistesleben Stuttgart (3rd edition 2016) / P. 53: provided by the State Archives of the Canton of Schwyz: Schweizerisches Archiv für Volkskunde, 15/1911, pp. 89–94, 177–184 / p. 81 © Eduardo Saiz Alonso / p. 120 Chang, S. et al. (2017): "Nutri tional composition and heavy metal content of the human placenta". In: *Placenta* 60: 100–102.

Printed in Poland
by Amazon Fulfillment
Poland Sp. z o.o., Wrocław

51800033R00105